Nursing and Family Caregiving
Social Support and Nonsupport

Anne Neufeld, RN, PhD, is a Professor in the Facility of Nursing at the University of Alberta, Edmonton, Canada. She teaches in public health nursing, aging, and nursing research. Her research focuses on family caregiving and social support and nonsupport for women and men family cargivers, support for family caregivers of seniors with chronic conditions, immigrant women caregivers' experience of support, and multicultural meanings of social support among immigrants and refugees. She has pulished research and methodological articles in journals such as the *Canadian Journal on Aging,* the *Canadian Journal of Nursing Research,* the *Journal of Advanced Nursing,* the *Journal of Family Nursing, Public Health Nursing,* and *Qualitative Health Research.* Based on a shared background in public health nursing and a common interest in social support, she and Dr. Harrison have collaborated for over 20 years on a program of research addressing social support among family caregivers. Their exploration of support in diverse family caregiving situations has been faicilitated by their focus on different populations in nursing; Dr. Neufeld's focus is on older adults, and Dr. Harrison's focus is families with infants and toddlers.

Margaret J. Harrison, PhD, is a Professor Emeritus in the Facility of Nursing at the University of Alberta, where she taught family theory and research and community health nursing. She was the recipient of a Medical Research Council Health Scholar Award. Her research addresses families with children and family caregivers. She has collaborated for over 20 years with Dr. Neufeld on studies that address social support for family caregivers. In addition, her research examined mother and father interactions with infants and toddlers and has included an intervention study with fathers of infants. She has published research and methodological articles in journals such as *Research in Nursing & Health, Qualitative Health Research, Health Care for Women International, Public Health Nursing,* the *Journal of Advanced Nursing,* and the *Canadian Journal of Nursing Research.*

Nursing and Family Caregiving

Social Support and Nonsupport

ANNE NEUFELD, RN, PhD

MARGARET J. HARRISON, PhD

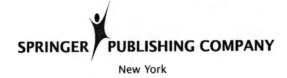

SPRINGER PUBLISHING COMPANY

New York

Springer Publishing Company, LLC
11 West 42nd Street
New York, NY 10036
www.springerpub.com

Acquisitions Editor: Allan Graubard
Project Manager: Megan Washburn
Cover Design: Mimi Flow
Composition: Publication Services, Inc.

E-book ISBN: 978-0-8261-1130-2

10 11 12 13/5 4 3 2 1

Printed in the United States of America by Offset Paperback Manufacturers

The authors and the publisher of this Work have made every effort to use sources believed to be reliable to provide information that is accurate and compatible with the standards generally accepted at the time of publication. Because medical science is continually advancing, our knowledge base continues to expand. Therefore, as new information becomes available, changes in procedures become necessary. We recommend that the reader always consult current research and specific institutional policies before performing any clinical procedure. The authors and publisher shall not be liable for any special, consequential, or exemplary damages resulting, in whole or in part, from the readers' use of, or reliance on, the information contained in this book. The publisher has no responsibility for the persistence or accuracy of URLs for external or third-party Internet Web sites referred to in this publication and does not guarantee that any content on such Web sites is, or will remain, accurate or appropriate.

Library of Congress Cataloging-in-Publication Data

Neufeld, Anne.
Nursing and family caregiving : social support and nonsupport / Anne Neufeld, Margaret Harrison.
    p. ; cm.
  Includes bibliographical references.
  ISBN 978-0-8261-1129-6 (alk. paper)
  1. Caregivers. 2. Home Nursing. I. Harrison, Margaret, 1941- II. Title.
  [DNLM: 1. Home Nursing--psychology. 2. Caregivers--psychology. 3. Emigrants and Immigrants--psychology. 4. Interpersonal Relations. 5. Research Design. 6. Social Support. WY 200 N482n 2009]
  RA645.3.N48 2009
  362.14--dc22

                                                        2009043447

To our families and to our colleagues
who have been important sources
of social support for us

Contents

Foreword

CONTRIBUTIONS OF QUALITATIVE INQUIRY
TO THE ANALYSIS OF SOCIAL SUPPORT

Social support is a concept that has been used extensively in research since it was introduced as a scientific concept by Caplan in 1974. It is an extremely *useful* concept, both for researchers exploring the interaction, caring, and helping behaviors during illness and disability, and for health professionals assessing patient and family needs.

The usage of social support has increased over the past four decades, and it will eventually find its way into the lay lexicon. But the increasing use of the term in research and professional literature is not without cost and may be confusing. It has led to modification and dispersion (Hupcey, 1998b) and subtle-changes in the meaning and use of the concept. In her analysis of the multiple uses of social support, Hupcey (1998a) noted that it is the various configurations of social support that have been modified over the years, and these changes in definition have resulted in confusion in the body of research literature. These changes in definitions were sometimes deliberate, but they often existed as inconsistencies between the operational definition of social support and how the concept was used in the study. For instance, social support was sometimes conceived as unidirectional, extending from the caregiver to the recipient, and was sometimes conceived as a two-way interaction, with reciprocity a part of the social support interaction. Sometimes the recipient had to be aware of the support for the interaction to be classified as *social support,* but sometimes not. These differences are important, because the outcomes of such projects cannot be easily compared and are difficult to synthesize.

The quantitative social support literature is international and voluminous; researchers have correlated social support with every imaginable health outcome and examined social support throughout the life span. Even patient deficits may be couched as social support *needs*. For instance, from quantitative inquiry, we know that the greater the *social support*, the lower the stigma concerns in those with HIV (Laros, Davis, Gallo, Heinrich, & Talavera, 2009). It is a predictor of maternal-fetal attachment (Yarcheski, Mahon, Yarcheski, Hanks, & Cannella, 2009). Parent support is a protective factor for children's development of post-traumatic stress disorder in war zones in Palestine (Thabet, Ibraheem, Shivram, Winter, & Voatanis, 2009). Women living with a partner are more likely to report with a smaller breast cancer lesion, either by locating it earlier, or from receiving support to seek treatment sooner than they would otherwise (Kricker et al., 2009). Other important considerations were differences in the types of social support provided by lay networks and whether professional support should be considered *social support* or whether it was a different type of support, such as obligatory support (Hupcey & Morse, 1998).

Despite this, the differences in types of support offered continue to be classified within broad categories, such as emotional, informational, instrumental, or financial (see Chapter 1). Yet these broad categories are problematic for practitioners, because this categorization lacks adequate details on the *mechanisms* and *meanings* of support for utilization. The literature does not show us *how* or *why* social support functions to make these differences.

Qualitative researchers have also published on social support, and this research provides the necessary microanalytic detail missing in quantitative inquiry. We have studied the nature of social support in health and illness. We have studied the abilities of patients to reciprocate and even considered whether social support existed if the recipient was unaware—or unconscious—when the support was provided.

To date, most of this qualitative research consists of single studies, conducted within a single context. As such, the research is fragmented and therefore not as useful as it might be. Hence, this volume contributes a much needed synthesis; it fills a huge void and can make a significant contribution to a cluttered and busy field.

Since 1995, Neufeld, Harrison, and their colleagues have been systematically conducting a series of qualitative studies on social support that target the lay or family caregiver as the recipient of support, rather than the support between the caregiver and the patient recipient. Their research program, consisting of 12 projects, explores the support requirements of lay caregivers in various contexts and with different populations. Thus this text is a truly amazing microanalytic compendium of social support strategies in different family configurations, in different contexts and ethnic groups, and filling different types of needs.

But the research does not stop there—the authors consider the initiators to and ramifications of social support, the nonsupportive interactions and the so-called side effects of too little or too much social support. They explore the process of access, of formal barriers to support, and even nonsupportive interactions. Is social support always positive? Can social support be disabling? When and under what conditions? Is reciprocation necessary? How does obligation occur? When?

Two unique aspects of this work should be noted. The first is the variety of qualitative methods used to elicit the participants' perspectives on caregiver support. Neufeld and Harrison's research moves beyond semistructured interviews, to use card sorts, to elicit characteristics, and network analyses: thus making the research both mixed- and multiple-method; a discussion of methods is provided for researchers following in their path.

The second important aspect of this work is its clinical application. The authors even include a clinical tool for assessment of social support (Chapter 8). Supporting the caregiver has been a priority in community health for several decades, and it is of great importance in the containment of health care costs. This volume makes a significant contribution to our understanding of family and caregiver functioning and how these caregiving networks may be utilized, strengthened, and understood.

Janice M. Morse

REFERENCES

Caplan, G. (1974). *Support systems and community mental health.* New York: Behavioral Publications.

Hupcey, J. (1998a). Clarifying the social support theory-research relationship. *Journal of Advanced Nursing, 27,* 1231–1241.

Hupcey, J. (1998b). Social support: Assessing conceptual coherence. *Qualitative Health Research, 8*(3), 304–318.

Hupcey, J., & Morse, J. M. (1998). Can a professional relationship be considered social support? *Nursing Outlook, 45*(6), 270–276.

Kricker, A., Price, M., Butow, P., Goumas, C., Armes, J. E., & Armstrong, B. K. (2009). Effects of life events and social support on the odds of a ≤ 2cm breast cancer. *Cancer Causes and Control, 20,* 437–447.

Laros, S. E, Davis, J. N., Gallo L. C., Heinrich, J., & Talavera, G. (2009). Concerns about stigma, social support and quality of life in low-income HIV-positive Hispanics. *Ethnicity & Disease 19*(1), 65–70.

Thabet, A. A., Ibraheem, A. N., Shivram, R., Winter, E. A., & Voatanis, P. (2009). Parenting support and PTSD in children of a war zone. *International Journal of Social Psychiatry, 55*(3), 226–237.

Yarcheski, A., Mahon, N. E., Yarcheski, T., Hanks, M. M., & Cannella, B. L. (2009). A meta-analytic study of predictors of maternal-infant attachment. *International Journal of Nursing Studies, 46*(5), 708–715.

Preface

Caring for a family member with a chronic health condition is an increasingly common experience. Nurses and other practitioners work with family caregivers and their families to facilitate support for family caregivers as they care for their dependent relatives. In this book, we present an integration of qualitative research findings for the use of nurses and other health and social care practitioners and researchers concerned with mobilizing support for individuals caring for an adult or child family member with a health condition. Findings were generated from a program of research on family caregiving and social support that was conducted over a number of years. In writing this book, we seek to address the demand for presentation of research findings, including those from qualitative research, as evidence for guidance in practice and for research that builds on existing knowledge and employs approaches for working with vulnerable populations.

Practitioners and researchers who may find this book useful include those working with families in settings such as long-term care, hospices, or oncology treatment facilities and professionals in community agencies working with families who care for adults, infants, or children with health issues or chronic conditions. The book provides insight into the experience of family caregivers and describes the impact of support. This information is valuable to practitioners and professionals who provide care and who plan programs or develop policies intended to assist family caregivers. Researchers whose focus is family work, family caregiving, or social networks and social support may also find the book informative.

Our presentation is derived from a within-program integration of findings across qualitative studies that examined a similar research question and were conducted by our research teams. Study participants included men and women caring for a relative or friend with a health condition and living in a large metropolitan area in Western Canada. We describe our viewpoint on working with family caregivers, as well as the theoretical perspectives that guided our research.

Family caregiving is a demanding responsibility that, in the absence of adequate support, may have a negative impact on caregivers' health. To meet caregiving demands, caregivers rely on social support from family and friends, as well as from professionals, but may also experience nonsupportive interactions and a lack of support. In this book, we provide illustrative examples of the supportive and nonsupportive interactions that men and women caregivers experienced and discuss the factors that influence their experience. Our focus then shifts to mobilization of social support, from the informal social network of kin and friends, and from formal, professional sources, including mobilization of support in the context of migration. Caregivers' advocacy for their relative in response to the experience of nonsupportive interactions is also described. We summarize our findings on social support and family caregiving and suggest key concepts to consider in working with family caregivers. For illustrative purposes, these concepts are applied to three potential caregiving scenarios.

Research conducted with a vulnerable population, such as family caregivers, requires approaches that recognize their vulnerability and provide caregivers with the supportive conditions to choose what they will share and to express their experience—in their own words in the setting of their choice. In the final section of the book, we have included a discussion of methodological approaches that we employed in our research program to address these challenges. These approaches may be useful for those who conduct research with similar populations.

The women and men who shared with us their experience in caring for a relative contributed experiential knowledge of the challenge of sustaining their role as family caregivers while they sought to provide the best possible care for their relative. It is our hope that this integrative presentation of their experience with support and nonsupport will be useful to practitioners and researchers who seek to facilitate support for family caregivers and will honor the contributions to our research made by family caregivers.

Anne Neufeld and Margaret J. Harrison

We wish to acknowledge with thanks the generosity of the women and men caregivers and their families who welcomed us warmly into their homes and willingly shared their time and their stories. We also recognize the contributions of professionals who have served as members of advisory teams for research studies and participated in focus group discussions.

Our thanks to our co-investigators and co-authors on the research publications that formed the basis for this book for their consistent and creative contributions to the research studies over the many months required to complete longitudinal qualitative research projects. We also thank our colleagues and former colleagues who have provided helpful feedback on our work.

Throughout our work on this program of research, we have received valuable assistance from many graduate students and from a postdoctoral fellow whose contributions we also wish to recognize.

We acknowledge with thanks funding for this program of research, which was provided by the following agencies listed in alphabetical order: Alberta Association of Registered Nurses Research Fund; Alberta Foundation for Nursing Research; Alzheimer Society of Canada; Canadian Institutes of Health Research; Caritas Foundation of Edmonton; Central Research Fund, University of Alberta; Social Sciences and Humanities Research Council of Canada through the Prairie Centre of Excellence for Research on Immigration and Integration at the University of Alberta; University of Alberta Support for Advancement of Scholarship program.

Nursing and Family Caregiving

Social Support and Nonsupport

The Experience of Family Caregiving: Social Support and Nonsupport

Care of a family member with a health condition is a common experience that can be challenging for family caregivers as well as for practitioners who work with families. An understanding of the interactions that family caregivers experience can assist practitioners and researchers in avoiding actions or suggestions that family caregivers view as nonsupportive despite the professionals' intention to be supportive. In Part 1 of this book, we present findings from our program of research on family caregiving and social support with men and women family caregivers who are assisting vulnerable adults or children with a health condition. We suggest a sensitizing framework that can guide professional approaches to facilitating support for family caregivers and research on family caregiving and social support.

We begin in Chapter 1 with a presentation of the background perspectives that guided us, including a framework for presentation of our research findings and a discussion of the application of qualitative research to practice. Our framework incorporates personal and social factors influencing the experience of supportive and nonsupportive interactions as well as caregivers' perceptions of the consequences of these interactions.

The remaining chapters in this section were written to be read either in sequence or in the order of most interest to the reader. In Chapters 2 to 5, we present our findings on supportive and nonsupportive interactions; the approaches that family caregivers used in monitoring, reflecting, and mobilizing support from kin and friends or from professional sources; and discuss different perspectives on the intersection of support from the social networks of kin and friends as well as professionals. The impact of migration and culture on family caregivers' ability to obtain support is outlined in Chapter 6. Some caregivers become a strong advocate for their relative in response to the experience of nonsupportive interactions, which is described in Chapter 7.

To conclude Part I, in Chapter 8 we discuss the application of our research findings to practice. This chapter incorporates suggestions on how health care professionals may use the framework we identified as a guide to facilitate support of family caregivers.

1   Caregiving and Social Support

Most of us know someone who is providing care to a family member with a health condition. This common responsibility includes many challenges for family caregivers (Kim & Schulz, 2008; Sullivan-Bolyai, Deatrick, Gruppuso, Tamborlane, & Grey, 2003). The growing numbers of older individuals with chronic illness or disability, and the increasing number of children with chronic conditions such as diabetes, have expanded the involvement of family members as primary caregivers for a relative. Family caregivers—most of whom are women, although caregiving by men is increasing—may be juggling their care of a relative with employment outside the home and be vulnerable to health impacts such as depression (Cannuscio et al., 2004). In addition, family caregiving may present economic burdens, related to costs of care and reduced employment (Kim & Schulz, 2008). These demands are accentuated in a societal context in which changes in health care delivery for conditions such as cancer have reduced the length of hospital stays and increased the health care system's expectation of family participation in care of relatives (Kim & Schulz, 2008).

Individuals caring for family members rely on support from family and friends, as well as support from professionals, while meeting the demands of caregiving (Raina et al., 2004). They may, however, experience nonsupportive interactions and a lack of support from family, friends, and health professionals, or make limited use of resources

3

available to them in their community (Neufeld & Harrison, 2003). In the absence of adequate support, caregiving demands can have a negative impact on the health of caregivers and may limit their ability to continue to care for their relative (Raina et al., 2004).

Nurses and other health and social care practitioners, as well as researchers studying family caregiving and social support, require an understanding of the supportive and nonsupportive interactions that family caregivers experience. Practitioners can incorporate these dimensions in their assessment of the support needs and resources of a caregiver, and researchers can build on these insights in designing research studies. In addition, information on nonsupportive interactions can assist professionals in avoiding actions or suggestions that caregivers view as nonsupportive—even when the approaches used by professionals are intended to be supportive.

In this book we present findings from our program of research on family caregiving and social support. On the basis of these findings, we suggest a sensitizing framework to guide professional approaches to facilitating support for family caregivers and research on family caregiving and social support.

GUIDING PERSPECTIVES ON FAMILY CAREGIVING

Within nursing and other health professions such as medicine, it is usually an individual with a health problem who is the patient or the primary focus of care. Family members who assist the ill individual are unlikely to be the focus of intervention except when health professionals make an effort to guide them on how to give the required assistance to their relative, such as administering medication, preparing appropriate diets, or assisting with prescribed exercise. The traditional focus of professionals on individuals with a health problem, shown schematically in Figure 1.1 as overlapping circles representing the individual and the health professional, overlooks the presence of the social network of the dependent individual with the health problem (portrayed in the third circle) and the care and support the individual receives from family and friends.

From a clinical perspective Christakis (2004) argued that we need to include consideration of the social networks of patients in planning and giving care. We agree with Christakis that nurses and other health and social care professionals should be attentive to the role of family caregivers and friends who provide care in community settings for adults and

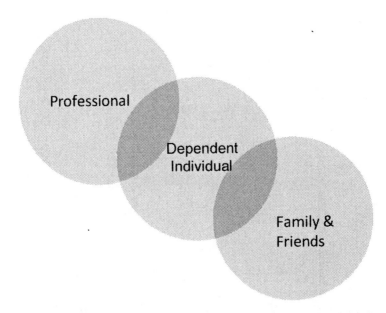

Figure 1.1. Professionals' focus on an individual dependent client with a health problem.

children with health conditions. We view family caregivers as an important component of an individual's social network. In Figure 1.2 we portray health care professionals, family caregivers, and the individual with a health problem as overlapping circles with areas of mutual concern.

Family care for ill and dependent family members provides benefits for both the ill individual and the caregiver and may reduce the social costs of care, but there is the potential for a negative impact on the health and functioning of family caregivers. From the perspective of nurses and other professionals working in community settings, it is evident that the demands of family caregiving can exact a toll on the health and functioning of family caregivers. In Figure 1.3, we added a fourth circle to include consideration of the social network of family and friends, who are current or potential sources of support for the family caregiver.

We believe that an understanding of the support that is available to family caregivers assists those professionals who interact with them, enabling the professional to work with clients and their family caregivers to sustain support. Recently the work of other researchers also has focused on the support available to family caregivers from their informal and formal social networks (Charlesworth, Tzimoula, Higgs,

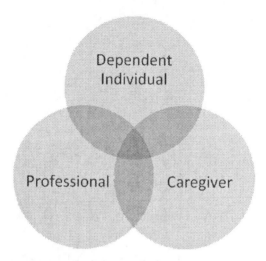

Figure 1.2. Professionals' inclusion of the family caregiver with the dependent individual.

& Poland, 2007; Hart et al., 2007) acknowledging the importance of support in assisting the caregiver to provide aid. Before presenting our research findings, we would like to provide some background in this introductory chapter to our research program and the issue of family caregiving. We begin the chapter with a brief scenario representative of the caregiving situations in our research program. The scenario is a composite based on individuals we interviewed. We then describe the theoretical concepts that informed our research on support for family caregivers, in particular, concepts of social networks and social exchange theory. We next provide an overview of the findings from our research program on family caregivers' experience of support, which was guided by the theoretical concepts presented. We conclude the chapter by addressing the contribution of qualitative research to clinical practice and present our argument that the findings of our research program meet the criteria for potential use in clinical practice

FAMILY CAREGIVING SCENARIO

Our research has included family caregivers in varied caregiving situations. Although there were variations in the medical conditions of their relatives, we learned that the experience of caregivers in accessing

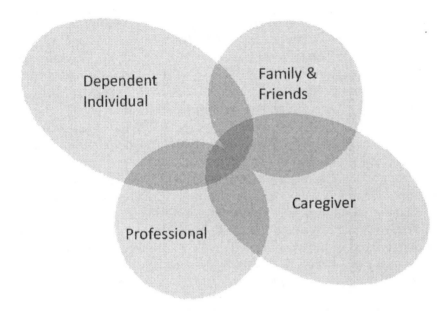

Figure 1.3. Professionals' inclusion of the family caregiver and the network of family and friends with the dependent individual.

support was similar. We constructed the following scenario to incorporate aspects of the caregiving experience that were frequently encountered in our research. Following the scenario, we suggest several questions in relation to this situation for you to consider while reading the subsequent chapters in the book.

> For 5 years, Mary has cared at home for her husband, who has Alzheimer's disease, high blood pressure, and diabetes. Her husband no longer recognizes her. He requires assistance with washing, dressing, and eating; is confused in unfamiliar situations; and often tries to leave the house without her. Although Mary has three adult children in the city, she and her husband live by themselves. She would like her children to spend more time assisting in the care of her husband because her health is poor. However, her children are busy in their work and have suggested placing their father in a nursing home. Mary is angry at this suggestion; she would like to get more services for her husband so that she can continue to care for him at home. However, she is not sure where to begin and feels overwhelmed with the daily demands of caregiving and her husband's need for constant supervision.

We encourage the reader to reflect on several questions in relation to Mary's situation as a context for reading the subsequent chapters. The questions include: What are Mary's struggles? What are her resources? What would be helpful to Mary beyond what she already has? From whom could she get help (e.g., family, friends, professionals, community resources)? How might she mobilize these resources? What circumstances could affect her ability to access aid? What changes in the resources available in your community might be needed to assist Mary? What changes in policy might be required to assist her? These questions highlight areas that we addressed in our research, such as the experience of supportive and nonsupportive interactions while caregiving, and the mobilization of support from family, friends, and professionals.

To provide a background for the discussion of our research on social support and caregiving, we next outline the role of social support in family caregiving and health. This section also includes a summary of major theoretical concepts in social network and social exchange theory.

FAMILY CAREGIVING, HEALTH, AND SOCIAL SUPPORT

Care for relatives with a health condition occurs throughout the life span and includes both women and men (Navaie-Waliser, Spriggs, & Feldman, 2002). Although in the past most family caregivers were women, the gap between the number of women and men caregivers, including those caring for older relatives, is narrowing (Swanberg, Kanatzar, Mendiondo, & McCoskey, 2006). Psychological outcomes to which family caregivers are particularly vulnerable include depression and stress. Older caregivers, those with low economic status, and those with a limited support network are especially vulnerable, and situations involving care of a relative with dementia or cancer may be particularly challenging (Kim & Schulz, 2008; Schulz & Sherwood, 2008). In a U.S. survey of a nationally representative sample of informal caregivers, including relatives and friends of older persons with cancer, dementia, diabetes, or frailty, men and women caring for someone with cancer or dementia reported greater levels of psychological distress and physical strain than those caring for someone with diabetes or frailty (Kim & Schulz, 2008). There may be differences between men and women caregivers in the effect of caregiving on their health. Women, in comparison to men caregivers, experience poorer emotional health, are less likely to use respite services, but may increase participation in religious activities (Navaie-Waliser et al., 2002). In another study (Calasanti & King, 2007), men caring for a spouse with dementia reported increased use of alcohol and antidepressants as well as the use of coercion with their spouse in an effort to cope with their stress. To our knowledge, the use of alcohol and coercion as coping strategies has not been examined in studies of women family caregivers.

Social support is linked to health (Berkman, Glass, Brissette, & Seeman, 2000; Cohen, 2004; Smith & Christakis, 2008) and may enhance the ability of family caregivers to sustain their role as caregivers for child or adult relatives as support levels often diminish during caregiving (Kiecolt-Glaser, Dura, Speicher, Trask, & Glaser, 1991). With respect to parents, a review of literature indicates that parents caring for children with cancer are at risk for negative emotional and physical health outcomes and that limited social support is a risk factor for negative psychological outcomes, particularly for mothers (Rabineau, Mabe, & Vega, 2008). Among caregivers of a relative with dementia, a 5-year longitudinal study found that higher levels of satisfaction with social support were associated with fewer symptoms of depression (Clay, Roth, Wadley, & Haley, 2008).

THE ROLE OF SOCIAL NETWORKS AND RELATIONSHIPS IN ACCESS TO SOCIAL SUPPORT

Social Network

A social network refers to a set of actors, or group of individuals, and the relationship ties among them (Felmlee, 2003). The nature of the social network composition and the quality of the family caregivers' connections with members of their network can influence their access and potential access to supportive interactions. Social network ties can vary in terms of the number of persons in the network, density or interconnections among network members, and homogeneity or the degree of similarity among members of the network (Carpentier & Ducharme, 2005). For example, a woman caring for her husband might have a social network consisting of her two adult children and a neighbor. Her network would be described as small (3 people), dense (her son and daughter are also friends of the neighbor, and they interact often), and homogeneous (all members of the social network share similar ethnic, economic, and religious characteristics). In comparison, a mother caring for a child with severe asthma might have a social network consisting of her husband, her mother, three sisters, and two friends from church, as well as multiple contacts among her coworkers in a store (5) and members of her yoga group (12) at her fitness club. This social network would be described as large (24) and heterogeneous, with loose connections among some members.

Caregivers have connections to health professionals, as well as to family and friends, and rely on these connections or social ties for assistance in meeting family caregiving demands (Carpentier & Ducharme, 2003). There are different theoretical perspectives on how informal (family and friends) and formal (professional and community agencies) sources interact in providing support through time and in relation to variations in caregiving demands. However, there is consensus on the importance of social ties as a source of social support. Other research has addressed social networks and preferences for family or professional sources (Carpentier & Ducharme, 2003, 2005; Sin, 2006). Typologies of support networks have identified variations in support available within the context of different types of social networks (Wenger, 1991). As an illustration of preferences in types and sources of support, the first woman whose social network was described previously may prefer to receive help from her daughter in giving personal care to her husband but seek support from her son for financial matters and go to her neighbor when she wants a respite from supervising her husband so that she can go out to a movie. She is likely to prefer support from family members (informal network) rather than from social or health care agencies (formal network). This family caregiver may access home care assistance from the local health care agency only when she can no longer cope with the caregiving demands and develops health issues of her own.

Social Exchange Theory

The nature of relationships among members of the social network is important for support. Social exchange was defined by Homans (1961) as the exchange of activity, tangible or intangible, and rewarding or costly, between at least two people. One of the propositions of social exchange theory is that behavior has both costs and rewards; in general, behavior that is rewarded is likely to be repeated. Social exchange also involves the principle that when an individual assists another, there is a general expectation of some reciprocation or return in the future, although the reciprocation might not be stipulated in advance (Blau,

1986, p. 93). Over the past two decades, research in social psychology using social exchange theory has differentiated between negotiated exchanges and reciprocal exchanges (Cook & Rice, 2003).

Negotiated exchanges involve the division of a finite pool of resources. Some individuals might have more control over valued resources than others, and consequently they have more power in a relationship, even if they are unaware of it (Cook & Emerson, 1978). From this theoretical perspective, discussions that home care nurses have with family members over the type and amount of services that they can provide a client could be described as negotiated exchanges. In contrast, reciprocal exchanges are viewed as a process of "gift giving," or the giving of a valued resource or service that, with repetition over time, develops into an exchange relationship (Molm, Peterson, & Takahashi, 1999; Molm, Quist, & Wisely, 1994). Both partners in the relationship can provide rewards. From this perspective, a relationship will deteriorate when there is infrequent exchange of support. Power is not tied to access to resources, as in negotiated exchanges, but involves punitive sanctions or negative outcomes on the other. Relationships that develop over time between neighbors as they assist each other with everyday activities such as child care, transportation, social contact, or emotional support can be described as reciprocal exchanges. If one partner cannot or decides not to reciprocate, then the friendship will diminish over time.

Reciprocity is one dimension of the social network that has been addressed in research on family caregiving and is viewed as important to the ability of a caregiver to sustain caregiving while maintaining caregiver's social relationships. For example, some research indicates that there is more likelihood of exchanges of various forms of giving and receiving support between adult children and parents when there is a history of a positive relationship between the generations (Parrot & Bengston, 1999). Other research indicates that family caregivers can experience difficulty in maintaining reciprocity with family and friends and may experience restrictions in their relationships as a result of the demands of caregiving in situations such as care of a relative with dementia (Bunting, 1989). In addition, the potential for reciprocity within the caregiving relationship itself is limited when the care recipient is unable to communicate (Graham & Bassett, 2006; Neufeld & Harrison, 1995).

Reciprocity is important in the ability of a caregiver to sustain supportive relationships, as social exchange theory predicts that inequitable (nonreciprocal) exchanges will result in termination of relationships with associated loss of potential for support (Langford, Bowsher, Maloney, & Lillis, 1997). When there is no perceived opportunity to reciprocate social support, individuals may experience indebtedness (Greenberg & Westcott, 1983) and be less comfortable in the relationship. Inability to reciprocate or respond supportively can lead to perceptions of loss of independence, diminished self-worth, anger, and guilt (Roberto & Scott, 1986). For example, a man caring for his wife who has dementia might withdraw from social contacts with his friends at golf, not just because of the demands of caregiving on his time, but also because he is no longer able to participate in car pooling to the golf course or be on the planning committee for golf events.

A social exchange perspective has utility in guiding examination of relationships and interactions among members of a social network that are perceived as supportive or nonsupportive. However, examination of contextual influences such as culture or gender is also needed to facilitate understanding of the specific considerations individuals take into account as they evaluate the nature of their social interactions (Miller & Bermudez, 2004). For example, social and cultural expectations can influence the value placed on work done by men and women. A woman who assists her neighbor with house cleaning or meal preparation may be viewed as fulfilling an expected role, but may receive increased recognition and praise as a source of support when she shovels snow or repairs the fence. In this example, the latter activities are usually done by men in her social environment, and her actions are more highly valued when she crosses gender expectations.

Social Support

Extensive literature on social support addresses the concept from divergent perspectives, including distinctions between an individual's perception of receiving support, an observer's perspective that support was received, and a provider's perspective that support was given (Dunkel-Schetter, Blasband, Feinstein, & Herbert, 1992). Perceptions of support may be further differentiated as support that is available, used, or conflicted (Barrera, 1981; Barrera & Baca, 1990). Qualities of relationships and interactions in which support is experienced, such as intimacy and attachment, have also been identified as important

(Berkman, Glass, Brissette, & Seeman, 2000). The forms of support have been categorized in varied ways, such as instrumental, emotional, or informational (Cohen, 2004; Dunkel-Schetter, Folkman, & Lazarus, 1987; Langford et al., 1997) or as instrumental and financial, informational, appraisal, and emotional support (Berkman, et al., 2000).

In our research, we focused on the perspective of a recipient of support (Funch, Marshall, & Gebhardt, 1986), that is, the perspective or evaluation by a family caregiver that the content of social interactions was supportive. We included any type of support mentioned by the caregiver, including emotional, physical, and informational. We chose to focus on the caregivers' evaluations of the interactions they experienced because recipients' perceptions of social support may be one mechanism associated with long-term health effects of support (Berkman et al., 2000). However, not all interactions are supportive, and the caregiver's perception that interactions are nonsupportive may also have an important influence on health.

Nonsupportive Interactions

Parallel to our definition of support, we defined nonsupportive interactions as interactions and behaviors that are evaluated as unhelpful by caregivers within the context of their social interactions (Funch et al., 1986) with kin or friends (informal social network) and professionals or organizations (formal social network). Our definition included the understanding that nonsupportive interactions occur in the context of caregivers' relationships that are also sources of support (Neufeld & Harrison, 2003).

Studies of everyday relationships that do not include caregiving have identified numerous types of nonsupportive interactions. For example, Rook and colleagues (Rook, 1992, 2001; Rook & Pietromonaco, 1987) reported negative exchanges, invasion of privacy, and ineffective or excessive helping as nonsupportive interactions. Other types of nonsupportive interactions identified include conflict (Canary, Cupach, & Messman, 1995) and unwelcome advice, incurred obligation, and broken promises (Foa & Foa, 1980). Discouraging expression of emotion, hiding information, or consuming material resources (Malone, 1988; Wortman & Lehman, 1985) have also been reported as nonsupportive. Miscarried helping, which refers to efforts intended to help but perceived as unhelpful (Coyne, Wortman, & Lehman, 1988), is another form of non-supportive interaction.

Less information is available on nonsupportive interactions in caregivers' relationships, although this concept was included in our research. In interactions with family and friends, women caring for a relative with dementia experienced nonsupportive interactions in the form of unmet expectations and negative interactions (Neufeld & Harrison, 2003). Unmet expectations occurred when potential helpers offered assistance but did not follow through, failed to maintain expected social contact, offered assistance that was a poor fit with the caregivers' needs, or lacked the ability to provide help. Negative interactions took the form of disparaging comments about the caregiver, conflict over appraisal of the care recipient's health status, and spillover of longstanding family conflicts.

In relationships with professionals, family caregivers' experience of nonsupportive interactions may include disagreement about help needed, difficulty in obtaining a satisfactory quality of aid, or problems monitoring services that are provided (Hasselkus, 1988). Lack of cultural sensitivity is an additional form of nonsupportive interaction experienced particularly by immigrant caregivers (Neufeld, Harrison, Stewart, Hughes, & Spitzer, 2002). Stewart and colleagues studied caregiving situations, including care of children with chronic conditions, adults with hemophilia or HIV/AIDS, and seniors with stroke (Stewart, 2000; Stewart, Hart, & Mann, 1995; Stewart, Ritchie, McGrath, Thompson, & Bruce, 1994). They found absent support, miscarried helping, conflicted interactions, inadequate reciprocity, stressful interactions, and negative interactions such as prejudice, uncertainty, and loss of confidentiality. Although limited, information indicates the presence of several forms of nonsupportive interactions in the relationships of family caregivers with their family and friends as well as professionals.

Conditions Influencing Perceptions of Support

Berkman and colleagues (2000) have proposed a comprehensive model for the study of social support that incorporates "upstream" social conditions that influence support, including the composition of social networks, psychosocial experiences of support, and pathways that may be influential for health (Berkman et al., 2000). They argue that social conditions such as culture, socioeconomic factors, public policies, and political culture, as well as social changes, are structural conditions that influence and shape both social network structures and the characteristics of network ties. They have suggested that these upstream factors provide opportunities for the "downstream" psychosocial experience of support, social influence, social interactions and relationships, and access to resources that ultimately affect health through behavioral, psychological, and physiological pathways. Recognition of the complexity of structural and personal factors influencing support and the impact of support on health can facilitate our understanding of family caregivers' experience, including perceptions of barriers and nonsupportive interactions.

OUR PROGRAM OF RESEARCH

In this volume we present an integrative perspective of the findings from our research program on social support and family caregivers. We chose the term *integrative perspective* for specific reasons. We argue that integration of findings is appropriate for studies within our program of research, as all were guided by a common theoretical perspective and conducted by the same core team of researchers. Although we have focused on the integration of study findings that we have previously reported in journal articles and conference presentations, we also returned to the original data to obtain additional sample quotations or to confirm details about the participants or the concept discussed. We have analyzed the study findings for similarities and differences across the studies and identified concepts that could provide explanations for the body of our research as a whole. We employ the term *integrative perspective*, as we did not combine data from our studies and did not undertake new analyses of the original data. Reanalysis of data from combined studies has been termed qualitative secondary analysis (Sandelowksi & Barroso, 2007). The type of within-research program synthesis we used has been described as a borderline project, lying between qualitative secondary analysis and metasynthesis, which examines findings across qualitative studies from various research programs.

One of the requirements for any integration of research findings is that the studies examine a similar research question. The studies within our research program fit that requirement, as all studies included individuals who were caring for a family member or close friend with a health issue, and the study questions addressed their experience of supportive or nonsupportive interactions while giving care. The theoretical perspective of symbolic interaction (Blumer, 1967, 1969; Prus, 1996; Stryker, 1967) was the underlying framework guiding the design of all studies, which employed primarily an ethnographic approach in the sociological tradition (Hammersley & Atkinson, 1995). This theoretical perspective fit the background of the members of the research teams. We (coauthors) have a background in nursing, but our research collaborators included researchers from sociology and anthropology. All members of the research teams had interests in community health care, family work, and the use of critical perspectives to examine the experience of family caregivers.

A key assumption of symbolic interaction (Blumer, 1967, 1969; Prus, 1996; Stryker, 1967) is that human behavior evolves through a process of continuous interaction with others. From this perspective, individuals' perceptions and actions are understood within social and structural settings that are a source of power and control. This approach was useful for design of this research, as it facilitated understanding of the social context within which family caregivers function and perceive interactions as supportive or nonsupportive. We examined family caregiving and support in caregiving situations that included variations in conditions such as age, gender, immigration, adult or child care recipient, and care recipient diagnosis.

An implication of the use of an ethnographic approach informed by symbolic interaction was the importance of multiple contacts and sources of data generation. Our research studies included a range of data generation strategies, such as in-depth interviews with caregivers and other friends or family who assisted them, and focus group discussions with caregivers and professionals. Most frequently, we interviewed family caregivers several times in depth and asked them open-ended questions about their experience and perceptions. We also interviewed family caregivers in groups using focus group methods, observed them during their daily routine, and asked them to complete card sorts based on statements from earlier interviews while talking aloud to the researcher about their thoughts and decisions in sorting the cards. To supplement our understanding of the experience of family caregivers, we collected policy documents related to health and social services and diaries from family caregivers. The interview and focus group data, observations, and diaries were analyzed for themes and linkages among themes. The results of the card sort exercise were used to develop a taxonomy of behaviors in supportive and nonsupportive interactions.

Data analysis was primarily thematic and incorporated data segments from all sources that pertained to common ideas. Initial analysis involved descriptions of key ideas in words as close to those of the caregivers as possible. Subsequently, we identified linkages and patterns among key ideas. When research findings are integrated, information about the characteristics of the study participants enables nurses or other health care practitioners and researchers to understand the conditions under which the findings were generated and to identify the types of clients for whom the findings might be relevant.

In the chapters that follow, we present our research in relation to these dimensions of the support process. All the studies were conducted in a large metropolitan area in western Canada between 1988 and 2007 and included caregivers in varied caregiving situations. The study participants were men and women caring for a family member or close friend with a diagnosed health concern. Adult care recipients had cancer or dementia, and the family caregiver was either the adult child or spouse/partner of the person for whom they cared. Children who were care recipients had prematurity, asthma, or diabetes and were cared for by their mothers. Most of the interviews were conducted in English; a small number were done in Mandarin, Cantonese, Urdu, or Hindi. One of the studies specifically addressed the experience of immigrant women in providing family caregiving. In Table 1.1 we present a summary of the research studies included and the characteristics of the participants in each study.

The research studies were conducted during a period of reorganization in health care services involving an implied policy of increased reliance on family in the community to provide care for individuals facing chronic or acute health issues. Although the studies do address a variety of conditions, such as gender of the family caregiver, family role of the caregiver, and health condition and age of the care recipient, the integrative perspective presented in this book has some limitations. The data reflect the experience of family caregivers living in a country with basic medical care and hospitalization insurance provided by the government. Excluded from the studies were family caregivers for individuals with other chronic health concerns, such as multiple sclerosis or cardiovascular disease.

In Figure 1.4 we present an overview of the experience of family caregivers that was derived from the integration of findings from our program of research on social support. The core components of the process, as indicated within the circle, include the processes of monitoring and reflecting in relation to support demands and potential resources, and the process of mobilizing support from kin or friends as well as professional sources.

Table 1.1

CHRONOLOGICAL SUMMARY OF INCLUDED RESEARCH STUDIES AND STUDY PARTICIPANTS IN RESEARCH ON SOCIAL SUPPORT AND CAREGIVING

	PURPOSE	PARTICIPANT CHARACTERISTICS			
Publication		Number	Age range	Gender	Care recipient
Harrison, Neufeld, & Kusher, 1995	Support in life transitions	$n=11$	24–47 yrs.	F	Infant Child
Neufeld & Harrison, 1995	Reciprocity	$n=40$	25–71 yrs.	F	Elder with dementia; premature infant
Fudge, Neufeld, & Harrison, 1997	Support networks	$n=20$	37–71 yrs.	F	Elder with dementia
Harrison & Neufeld, 1997	Barriers to requesting aid	$n=40$	25–71 yrs.	F	Elder with dementia; premature infant
Neufeld & Harrison, 1998	Reciprocity & obligation	$n=22$	33–87 yrs.	M	Elder with dementia
Coe & Neufeld, 1999	Accessing formal support	$n=24$	33–87 yrs.	M	Elder with dementia
Neufeld, Harrison, Stewart, Hughes, & Spitzer, 2002	Migration, caregiving, connecting to resources	$n=29$	30–79 yrs.	F	Child with delayed development; adult with chronic condition
Heinrich, Neufeld, & Harrison, 2003	Strategies to interact with health personnel	$n=20$	37–71 yrs.	F	Elder with dementia
Neufeld & Harrison, 2003	Nonsupport from family and friends	$n=8$	30–79 yrs.	F	Elder with dementia
Spitzer, Neufeld, Harrison, Hughes, & Stewart, 2003	Migration, caregiving family, gender roles	$n=29$	30–79 yrs.	F	Child with delayed development; adult with chronic condition

Table 1.1

CHRONOLOGICAL SUMMARY OF INCLUDED RESEARCH STUDIES AND STUDY PARTICIPANTS IN RESEARCH ON SOCIAL SUPPORT AND CAREGIVING *(continued)*

	PURPOSE	PARTICIPANT CHARACTERISTICS			
Publication		**Number**	**Age range**	**Gender**	**Care recipient**
Neufeld, Harrison, Hughes, & Stewart, 2007	Nonsupportive interactions	*n*=59	19–72 yrs.	F	Premature infant; child with asthma, diabetes; adult with cancer; elder with dementia
Neufeld, Harrison, Hughes, & Stewart, 2007	Advocacy in response to nonsupport	*n*=34	19–72 yrs.	F	Premature infant; child with asthma, diabetes; adult with cancer; elder with dementia

Caregivers evaluated their experience within their relationships as supportive or nonsupportive and incorporated that interpretation into their ongoing monitoring and reflection. This process occurred within the context of influencing factors that included the caregiver's personal and cultural beliefs and expectations, migration, their informal social network of family and friends, their contact with the formal/professional social network, their caregiving situation, and their caregiving skills. Aspects of the informal network that were important influencing factors were the composition of the network, their location and the experience of migration, the provision of support for the caregiver's personal values, the receipt of offers of support, a history of reciprocity, and the experience of supportive or nonsupportive interactions in the caregiver's relationships with family and friends. The formal social network comprised health professionals, health care agencies, community groups, religious organizations, or government services. Aspects of the formal social network that were important influencing factors included composition of the network, location, policies influencing ease of access to services,

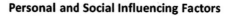

Personal and Social Influencing Factors

Personal & cultural beliefs & expectations   Migration
Informal social network   Formal/professional network
Caregiving situation   Caregiving skills

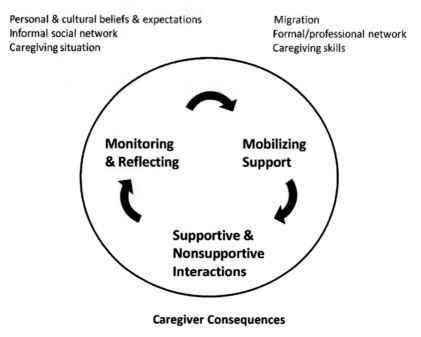

Caregiver Consequences

Feelings (positive, negative, mixed)   Personal growth/advocacy
Revised expectations & caregiver role   Changed or maintained social network

Figure 1.4. Caregivers' experience of social support.

support for the caregiver's personal beliefs and caregiving goals, mutuality, and supportive or nonsupportive interactions in their relationships with the caregiver. For the caregivers, the consequences of their experience in accessing support included a variety of positive, negative, or mixed feelings; revision of their expectations and role as a caregiver; personal growth in the form of becoming an advocate in response to nonsupportive interactions; and change in or maintenance of their social network ties.

Our goal in presenting this integration of findings from our program of research is to present findings in a form that will be useful for practitioners who work with family caregivers as well as researchers who study family caregiving and social support. Researchers may find integration of qualitative research findings in one volume a useful summary, and in Chapters 9 through 11 we discuss research issues that we addressed in the process of conducting research with vulnerable populations of family caregivers.

The contribution of qualitative research findings to practice has been a matter of recent interest, debate, and discussion. In the next section we present our perspective on the contribution of qualitative research to practice as background for readers who are practitioners.

CONTRIBUTION OF QUALITATIVE RESEARCH TO PRACTICE

The transfer of knowledge from research programs to clinical practice has received increasing emphasis in recent years. To achieve the best possible care for their clients, nurses and other health care professionals seek operating principles based on sound research to guide their practice. Two trends support the transfer of knowledge from research to practice: an accumulating body of findings from research programs that address questions of concern to practitioners, and increased emphasis on practice standards that promote evidence-based care.

Several challenges exist in transferring knowledge to practice, including the evaluation of research studies and the integration of knowledge across studies and research programs (Sandelowksi, 2004). One of the areas of difficulty has been the integration or synthesis of findings from qualitative research studies (Thorne, Jensen, Kearney, Noblit, & Sandelowski, 2004).

Qualitative research studies include the response of individuals to their health concerns and circumstances and a description of conditions under which variations occur in health issues. A goal of qualitative research is to generate an understanding, from the perspective of the participants, on questions such as: What are their responses to their health concerns over time? What is their explanation for why individual responses vary? What is their evaluation of the support they received from family, the community, and health care workers? A major contribution of qualitative research is this emphasis on in-depth understanding of individual experiences within the situational context. To obtain in-depth descriptions of individual experiences, a small number of individuals are interviewed, usually more than once, and the researcher might observe the participant in varied settings. Depending on the method used, the in-depth understanding generated may be presented as metaphors, themes with sample quotations, or a theoretical process with stages or a sequence over time.

The emphasis in qualitative research on conditions affecting an individual's response, the small sample sizes, the in-depth exploration of personal perspectives, and the varied format for presentation of findings have been obstacles to the integration of study findings. Some researchers have argued that the philosophical basis for qualitative work, which emphasizes individual experience, creates difficulties in integration of findings across studies, as metasynthesis of findings places distance between the reviewer doing the metasynthesis and the original participants. The difficulty in accurately representing the experience of others in reporting research findings has been described as a "crisis of representation" (Smith, 2004, pp. 962–963). However, other researchers have argued that it is possible to integrate findings from qualitative research (Sandelowski, 2006) if care is taken to describe the conditions under which the original findings were obtained while maintaining representational humility; that is, showing awareness of alternative readings or interpretations of the findings under investigation.

Researchers have addressed the contribution of qualitative research evidence for practice (Estabrooks, 1998; Morse, Hutchinson, & Penrod, 1998; Sandelowski, 1997, 2004) but in some cases hold divergent views. In this book, we consider the relevance of qualitative research evidence using the modes of clinical application suggested by Margaret Kearney (2001). She proposed that application of qualitative research evidence has four possibilities. Qualitative research evidence could contribute insight or empathy in understanding experience, provide detailed descriptive categories that can support development of new assessment tools, contribute information that could be shared with clients as a form of anticipatory guidance to assist them in anticipating what may be ahead in their experience, and provide a basis for coaching clients through sharing information about strategies that others in a similar situation may have used.

The potential utility of findings depends on the richness of detail, the extent to which findings are linked and interrelated, and the extent of the contextual information incorporated about familial, economic, social, environmental, or political contexts. Inclusion of detailed contextual information and insightful interpretation enhances the ability of clinicians to assess relevance of findings to a given situation. Clinicians play a major role in determining the strengths and limitations of peer-reviewed qualitative research evidence in relation to the setting in which they function and the personal characteristics and situations of the clients for whom they care.

OVERVIEW OF SUBSEQUENT CHAPTERS

In this chapter we presented background perspectives that guided our research program, including an introductory framework for presentation of our research findings as illustrated in Figure 1.4 and discussion of application of qualitative research to practice. Subsequent chapters are divided into two sections: Chapters 2 through 8 focus on presentation of an integration of the findings from our research studies and their application to practice, and the second section (Chapters 9 through 11) addresses issues in research.

Our findings on supportive interactions and relationship dimensions are discussed in Chapter 2, and in Chapter 3 we present findings on nonsupportive interactions experienced by caregivers in varied health situations. We then address the approaches that family caregivers used in monitoring, reflecting, and mobilizing support from kin and friends (Chapter 4) or from professional sources (Chapter 5). Also incorporated in Chapters 4 and 5 are discussions of varied perspectives on the intersection of support from these two social networks. In Chapter 6 we outline the impact of migration and culture on the ability of a family caregiver to obtain support. In several caregiving situations, caregivers described becoming advocates as a consequence of their experience of nonsupportive interactions, and this is described in Chapter 7.

Personal and social influencing factors are discussed throughout the chapters in the first section of the book. These chapters were written so that a reader could read them consecutively or in the order that is of most interest to them. The discussion of application of our research findings to practice is concentrated in Chapter 8. This chapter includes suggestions on how health care professionals may use the framework identified from our research as a guide to facilitate support of family caregivers.

Many health and social care practitioners and researchers work with vulnerable populations, such as family caregivers. In the final three chapters we describe approaches that enable individuals to tell their own story. These methods might be useful for nurses and others who conduct research in practice settings. Each chapter that focuses on research methods is a reprint of an article that has been previously published in a journal. We describe our use of inclusion of ecomaps and genograms in interviews to create a graphic portrayal of social networks (Chapter 9), our use of a card sort technique with think-aloud interviews to generate data in interviews and focus group discussions (Chapter 10), and the approaches we used to facilitate the participation of immigrant women in research (Chapter 11). All of these methods allow vulnerable individuals to choose what they will share with the researcher and express it in their words and in a setting of their choosing.

REFERENCES

Barrera, M. (1981). Social support in the adjustment of pregnant adolescents: Assessment issues. *Social Networks and Social Support, 4,* 69–96.

Barrera, M., & Baca, L. M. (1990). Recipient reactions to social support: Contributions of enacted support and network orientation. *Journal of Social and Personal Relationships, 7*(4), 541–551.

Berkman, L., Glass, T., Brissette, I., & Seeman, T. (2000). From social integration to health: Durkheim in the new millennium. *Social Science & Medicine, 51,* 843–857.

Blau, P. M. (1986). *Exchange and power in social life.* New Brunswick, NJ: Transaction.

Blumer, H. (1967). Society as symbolic interaction. In J. Manis (Ed.) *Symbolic interaction: A reader in social psychology* (pp. 139–148). Boston: Allyn & Bacon.

Blumer, H. (1969). *Symbolic interactionism.* Englewood Cliffs, NJ: Prentice Hall.

Bunting, S. (1989). Stress on caregivers of the elderly. *Advances in Nursing Science, 11*(2), 63–73.

Calasanti, T., & King, N. (2007). Taking "women's work" "like a man": Husbands' experiences of care work. *The Gerontologist, 47*(4), 516–527.

Canary, D., Cupach, W., & Messman, S. (1995). The nature of conflict in close relationships. In D. J. Canary, W. R. Cupach, & S. Messman (Eds.), *Relationship conflict in parent-child, friendship and romantic relationships* (pp. 1–21). Thousand Oaks, CA: Sage.

Cannuscio, C., Colditz, G., Rimm, E., Berkman, L., Jones, C., & Kawachi, I. (2004). Employment status, social ties, and caregivers' mental health. *Social Science & Medicine, 58,* 1247–1256.

Carpentier, N., & Ducharme, F. (2003). Care-giver network transformations: The need for an integrative experience. *Ageing & Society, 23,* 507–525.

Carpentier, N., & Ducharme, F. (2005). Support network transformations in the first stages of the caregiver's career. *Qualitative Health Research, 15*(3), 289–311.

Charlesworth, G., Tzimoula, X., Higgs, P., & Poland, F. (2007). Social networks, befriending and support for family carers of people with dementia. *Quality in Ageing: Policy, Practice and Research, 8*(2), 37–44.

Christakis, N. (2004). Social networks and collateral health effects [Editorial]. *British Journal of Medicine, 329,* 184–185.

Clay, O., Roth, D., Wadley, V., & Haley W. (2008). Changes in social support and their impact on psychosocial outcome over a 5-year period for African American and White caregivers. *International Journal of Geriatric Psychiatry, 23,* 857–862.

Coe, M., & Neufeld, A. (1999). Male caregivers' use of formal support. *Western Journal of Nursing Research, 2*(4), 568–588.

Cohen, S. (2004). Social relationships and health. *American Psychologist, 59*(8), 676–684.

Cook, K. S., & Emerson, R. M. (1978). Power, equity and commitment in exchange networks. *American Sociological Review, 43*, 721–739.

Cook, K. S., & Rice, E. (2003). Social exchange theory. In J. Delamater (Ed.), *Handbook of social psychology* (pp. 53–76). New York: Kluwer Academic/Plenum.

Coyne, J., Wortman, C. B., & Lehman, D. R. (1988). The other side of support: Emotional overinvolvement and miscarried helping. In B. H. Gottlieb (Ed.), *Marshalling social support formats, processes and effects* (pp. 305–331). Newbury Park, CA: Sage.

Dunkel-Schetter, C., Blasband, D., Feinstein, L., & Herbert, T. B. (1992). Elements of supportive interactions: When are attempts to help effective? In S. Spacapan, & S. Oskamp (Eds.), *Helping and being helped* (pp. 83–114). Newbury Park, CA: Sage.

Dunkel-Schetter, C., Folkman, S., & Lazarus, R. (1987). Correlates of social support receipt. *Journal of Personal and Social Psychology, 53*, 71–80.

Estabrooks, C. (1998). Will evidence-based practice make practice perfect? *Canadian Journal of Nursing Research, 30*(1), 15–36.

Felmlee, D. H. (2003). Interaction in social networks. In J. Delamater (Ed.), *Handbook of social psychology* (pp. 389–409). New York: Kluwer Academic/Plenum.

Foa, E. B., & Foa, U. G. (1980). Resource theory: Interpersonal behaviour as exchange. In K. J. Gergen, M. S. Greenberg, & R. H. Willis (Eds.), *Social exchange: Advances in theory and research* (pp. 77–94). New York: Plenum.

Fudge, H., Neufeld, A., & Harrison, M. H. (1997). Social networks of women caregivers. *Public Health Nursing, 14*(1), 20–27.

Funch, D. P., Marshall, J. R., & Gebhardt, G. P. (1986). Assessment of a short scale to measure social support. *Social Science & Medicine, 23*(3), 337–344.

Graham, J. E., & Bassett, R. (2006). Reciprocal relations: The recognition and co-construction of caring with Alzheimer's disease. *Journal of Aging Studies, 20*, 335–349.

Greenberg, M. S., & Westcott, D. R. (1983). Indebtedness as a mediator to reactions of aid. In J. D. Fisher, A. Nadler, & B. M. DePaulo (Eds.), *Recipient reactions to aid* (pp. 85–111). New York: Academic Press.

Hammersley, M., & Atkinson, P. (1995). *Ethnography: Principles in practice* (2nd ed.). London: Routledge.

Harrison, M. J., & Neufeld, A. (1997). Women's experience of barriers to support while caregiving. *Health Care for Women International, 18*, 591–602.

Harrison, M. J., Neufeld, A., & Kushner, K. (1995). Women in transition: Access and barriers to social support. *Journal of Advanced Nursing, 21*, 858–864.

Hart, T., O'Neil-Pirozzi, T. M., Williams, K. D., Rapport, L. J., Hammond, F., & Kreutzer, J. (2007). Racial differences in caregiving patterns, caregiver emotional function, and sources of emotional support following traumatic brain injury. *Journal of Head Trauma Rehabilitation, 22*(2), 122–131.

Hasselkus, B. R. (1988). Meaning in family caregiving: Perspectives on caregiver/professional relationships. *The Gerontologist, 28*, 686–691.

Heinrich, M., Neufeld, A., & Harrison, M. J. (2003). Seeking support: Caregivers' strategies for interacting with health personnel. *Canadian Journal of Nursing Research, 35*(4), 39–56.

Homans, G. C. (1961). *Social behavior and its elementary forms.* New York: Harcourt, Brace and World.

Kearney, M. (2001). Focus on research methods, levels and applications of qualitative research evidence. *Research in Nursing & Health, 24*, 145–153.

Kiecolt-Glaser, J., Dura, J., Speicher, C., Trask, J., & Glaser, R. (1991). Spousal caregivers of dementia victims: Longitudinal changes in immunity and health. *Psychosomatic Medicine, 53*, 345–362.

Kim, Y., & Schulz, R. (2008). Family caregivers' strains: Comparative analysis of cancer caregiving with dementia, diabetes, and frail elder caregiving. *Journal of Aging and Health, 20*(5), 483–503.

Langford, C. P. H., Bowsher, J., Maloney, J. P., & Lillis, P. P. (1997). Social support: A conceptual analysis. *Journal of Advanced Nursing, 25*(1), 95–100.

Malone, J. (1988). The social support social dissupport continuum. *Journal of Psychosocial Nursing, 26*(12), 18–22.

Miller, M. M., & Bermudez, J. M. (2004). Intersecting gender and social exchange theory in family therapy. *Journal of Feminist Family Therapy, 16*(2), 25–42.

Molm, L., Peterson, G., & Takahashi, N. (1999). Power in negotiated and reciprocal exchange. *American Sociological Review, 64*, 876–890.

Molm, L. D., Quist, T. M., & Wisely, P. A. (1994). Imbalanced structures, unfair strategies: Power and justice in social exchange. *American Sociological Review, 59*, 98–121.

Morse, J. M., Hutchinson, S. A., & Penrod, J. (1998). From theory to practice: The development of assessment guides from qualitatively derived theory. *Qualitative Health Research, 8*, 329–340.

Navaie-Waliser, M., Spriggs, M., & Feldman, P. (2002). Informal caregiving: Differential experiences by gender. *Medical Care, 40*, 1249–1259.

Neufeld, A., & Harrison, M. J. (1995). Reciprocity and social support in caregivers' relationships: Variations and consequences. *Qualitative Health Research, 5*, 348–365.

Neufeld, A., & Harrison, M. J. (1998). Men as caregivers: Reciprocal relationships or obligation? *Journal of Advanced Nursing, 28*(5), 959–968.

Neufeld, A., & Harrison, M. J. (2003). Unfulfilled expectations and negative interactions: Nonsupport in the relationships of women caregivers. *Journal of Advanced Nursing, 41*(4), 323–331.

Neufeld, A., Harrison, M. J., Hughes, K., & Stewart, M. (2007). Non-supportive interactions in the experience of women family caregivers. *Health and Social Care in the Community, 15*(6), 530–541.

Neufeld, A., Harrison, M. J., Stewart, M. J., Hughes, K. D., & Spitzer, D. (2002). Immigrant women: Making connections to community resources for support in family caregiving. *Qualitative Health Research, 14*(10), 1418–1428.

Parrott, T. M., & Bengston, V. L. (1999). The effects of earlier intergenerational affection, normative expectations and family conflict on contemporary exchanges of help and support. *Research on Aging, 21*, 73–105.

Prus, R. (1996). *Symbolic interaction and ethnographic research.* Albany: State University of New York Press.

Rabineau, K., Mabe, A., & Vega, R. (2008). Parenting stress in pediatric oncology populations. *Journal of Pediatric Hematology Oncology, 30*(5), 358–365.

Raina, P., McIntyre, C., Zhu, B., McDowell, I., Santaguida, L., Kristjansson, B., et al. (2004). Understanding the influence of the complex relationships among informal and formal supports on the well-being of caregivers of persons with dementia. *Canadian Journal on Aging, 23*(Suppl.), S43–S53.

Roberto, K. A., & Scott, J. P. (1986). Equity considerations in the friendships of older adults. *Journal of Gerontology, 41*, 241–247.

Rook, K. (1992). Detrimental aspects of social relationships: Taking stock of an emerging literature. In H. O. Veiel, & U. Baumann (Eds.), *The meaning and measurement of social support* (pp. 157–169). New York: Hemisphere.

Rook, K. (2001). Emotional health and positive versus negative exchanges: A daily diary analysis. *Applied Developmental Science, 5*(2), 86–97.

Rook, K., & Pietromonaco, P. (1987). Close relationships: Ties that heal or ties that bind. In D. Perlman & W. Jones (Eds.), *Advances in personal relationships* (pp. 1–35). Greenwich, CT: JAI.

Sandelowski, M. (1997). "To be of use": Enhancing utility of qualitative research. *Nursing Outlook, 45*(3), 125–132.

Sandelowski, M. (2004). Using qualitative research. *Qualitative Health Research, 14*(10), 1366–1386.

Sandelowski, M. (2006). "Meta-jeopardy": The crisis of representation in qualitative metasynthesis. *Nursing Outlook, 54*, 10–16.

Sandelowski, M., & Barroso, J. (2007). *Handbook for synthesizing qualitative research.* New York: Springer.

Schulz, R., & Sherwood, P. (2008). Physical and mental health effects of family caregiving. *American Journal of Nursing, 108*(9), 23–27.

Sin, C. (2006). Expectations of support among white British and Asian-Indian older people in Britain: The interdependence of formal and informal spheres. *Health & Social Care in the Community, 14*(3), 215–224.

Smith, J. K. (2004). Representation, crisis of. In M. S. Lewis-Beck, A. Bryman, & T. F. Liao (Eds.), *The Sage encyclopedia of social science research methods* (Vol. 3, pp. 962–963). Thousand Oaks, CA: Sage.

Smith, K., & Christakis, N. (2008). Social networks and health. *Annual Review of Sociology, 34*, 405–429.

Spitzer, D., Neufeld, A., Harrison, M. J., Hughes, K., & Stewart, M. J. (2003). "My wings have been cut, where can I fly?": Gender, migration and caregiving—Chinese and South Asian Canadian perspectives. *Gender and Society, 17*(2), 267–286.

Stewart M. J. (Ed.). (2000). *Chronic conditions and caregiving in Canada: Social support strategies.* Toronto, Canada: University of Toronto Press.

Stewart, M. J., Hart, J., & Mann, K. V. (1995). Living with hemophilia and HIV/AIDS: Support and coping. *Journal of Advanced Nursing, 22*(6), 1101–1111.

Stewart, M. J., Ritchie, J. A., McGrath, P., Thompson, D., & Bruce, B. (1994). Mothers of children with chronic conditions: Supportive and stressful interactions with partners and professionals regarding caregiving burdens. *Canadian Journal of Nursing Research, 26*(4), 61–82.

Stryker, S. (1967). Symbolic interaction as an approach to family research. In J. Manis (Ed.), *Symbolic interaction: A reader in social psychology* (pp. 371–383). Boston: Allyn & Bacon.

Sullivan-Bolyai, S., Deatrick, J., Gruppuso, P., Tamborlane, W., & Grey, M. (2003). Constant vigilance: Mothers' work parenting young children with type 1 diabetes. *Journal of Pediatric Nursing, 18*(1), 21–29.

Swanberg, J. E., Kanatzar, T., Mendiondo, M., & McCoskey, M. (2006). Caring for our elders: A contemporary conundrum for working people. *Families in Society: The Journal of Contemporary Social Services, 87*, 417–426.

Thorne, S., Jensen, L., Kearney, M., Noblit, G., & Sandelowski, M. (2004). Qualitative metasynthesis: Reflections on methodological orientation and ideological agenda. *Qualitative Health Research*, *14*(10), 1342–1365.

Wenger, G. C. (1991). A network typology: From theory to practice. *Journal of Aging Studies*, *5*(2), 147–162.

Wortman, C. B., & Lehman, D. R. (1985). Reactions to victims of life crises: Support attempts that fail. In I. G. Sarason & B. R. Sarason (Eds.), *Social support: Theory, research and applications* (pp. 463–489). Dordrecht, the Netherlands: Martinus Nijhoff.

2

Supportive Interactions, Reciprocity, and Obligation

The demands of caring for a relative with a health condition challenge a caregiver's personal and social resources and generate the need for assistance from others. Support is available to caregivers in the context of relationships with their friends and family, health professionals, and dependent relatives. However, family caregivers' experience of support may vary with their perceptions of reciprocity or obligation within those relationships. In this chapter we discuss the meaning of social support, particularly for women caregivers, and the relationship context of social support of women and men caregivers in interactions with others that include reciprocity and feelings of obligation.

In our research, we defined *social support* as the evaluation of the content of social interactions as helpful (Funch, Marshall, & Gebhardt, 1986). Our emphasis was on the perception of family caregivers, including the meaning of support for them, the types of support that they preferred and provided, and the key dimensions of the relationships within which they perceived support. Although social support can be examined from the perspective of the individual providing aid as well as the perspective of a bystander (Dunkel-Schetter, Blasband, Feinstein, & Herbert, 1992), we chose to give prominence to the family caregivers' evaluation of their interactions with others. We focused on their perception of support that might be available in their environment and their descriptions of supportive actions taken by family, friends, and health

29

professionals. As health professionals and researchers we were interested in understanding family caregivers' views of what was supportive, and communicating their perspective to other health care providers as a basis for improving the fit of the support and services that are provided.

We begin this chapter by describing interactions that family caregivers viewed as supportive. The meaning of support for women included emotional support, physical support, and informational support. After describing the meaning of support and providing illustrations of supportive interactions for each of these types of support, we describe the influence of the norm of reciprocity and the impact of belief in family obligations on the interactions of women and men family caregivers with the care recipient and others.

SUPPORTIVE INTERACTIONS

We explored the meaning of supportive interactions among women caregivers in diverse caregiving situations: women caring for an adult with cancer or an adult with dementia, mothers caring for infants born prematurely, and mothers caring for a child with asthma or diabetes (Neufeld, Harrison, Hughes, & Stewart, 2007). The descriptions of supportive interactions confirmed those of women who participated in one of our earlier studies (Harrison, Neufeld, & Kushner, 1995), a study that included mothers who were returning to work after an extended absence and mothers of new infants. Although mothers in this latter study experienced less intense caregiving demands, their descriptions add to our understanding of the social expectations that mothers and caregivers experience.

Women caregivers described the meaning of support in similar ways, although they were caring for individuals of different ages, with different health concerns, and different requirements for caregiving. Caregivers referred to emotional and physical support as well as information as a form of support. A woman caring for a relative with cancer described her perception of support in the following comments.

> Most of what I've been able to get is emotional. Someone to talk to you about . . . a problem, work through it. Someone who is willing to sit there and listen . . . Then there's physical support . . . It's good to have emotional support, you absolutely need that . . . But, support also means helping out because I can't handle it.

In their description of emotional support, women included their perception that support meant having someone to be a sounding board, to understand their experience, and to share their feelings as well as the load they carried while caregiving. It also meant getting feedback or appraisal from others, usually in the form of affirmation of the value of their work or new insight into their caregiving situation. Informational support meant having access to information and someone who could answer their questions. The words of a mother whose daughter had diabetes convey her desire for information.

> Someone who would listen to you first, and who would explain, not to a medical student, but you know, the ordinary man in the street language.

TYPES OF SUPPORT

Emotional Support

Women emphasized their experience of emotional support and elaborated on dimensions of emotional support such as being understood. A woman caring for a relative with dementia elaborated on having someone to talk to who could be a sounding board.

> Sometimes I need to talk something out so that I can find out what it exactly is that I need. Having people who are willing to listen, and then also having people who are willing to challenge it and say, "Yes, but what if . . ." or give me a little bit of different perspective. That's supportive for me.

Mothers in an earlier study expressed a similar idea.

> I just want someone to listen to me and to bounce ideas off of and to offer me some sort of objectivity which I'm unable to achieve.

A key dimension of emotional support was the perception by women caregivers that they were understood by family, friends, or health professionals. A woman caring for her grandmother with dementia describes how her coworkers understood her situation and her stress and allowed her to take time off.

> If I was crying they understood. They let me take time off. They were great.

A mother caring for an 18-year-old son with cancer described the experience of support as having others who understood as someone willing to share the load.

> Support is . . . to be there to help lift, but also to be there as a human being . . . to share your feelings too, to be a good support in the ups and downs. . . . The family support . . . like it's not just myself. I share the load with A. and my husband. So they understand.

Another key dimension of emotional support was appraisal of others, which occurred, for example, in the form of affirmation when they confirmed the value of the women's caring work, the personal demands that were involved in being a caregiver, and their insight into the nature of the caregiving role. For example, a woman who was caring simultaneously for her father with dementia, her mother who had advanced heart disease, and her husband who had several chronic conditions, including kidney failure, valued the appraisal in the form of affirmation of her caregiving that she received from her friends and her children:

> I get from my friends a lot, "I don't know how you do it. . . . You've got so much on your plate. How do you hold it together?" My kids keep coming to me and saying "You need to take some time for yourself."

Similarly, a woman who was the primary caregiver for a friend with cancer described how her daughter's appraisal in the form of affirmation was important for her,

> There were certain other things that E [her daughter] would say: "You know, Mom, you're doing a good job."

Other dimensions of emotional support were expressions of support that empowered them or provided advocacy for their relative, spiritual support, and respect for the caregiver that included maintaining confidentiality or privacy and respecting the caregiver's wishes. For example, parents of children with asthma or diabetes noted the importance of protection of their privacy; and trust was enhanced for mothers of infants or children or women caring for a relative with dementia when others openly acknowledged their errors. Possible errors included misjudgments in the treatment of the individual or misjudgments in how services were provided to their relative.

Physical Support

Although several women noted that emotional support was more often available to them, they valued practical aid when it was forthcoming. For example, a woman caring for her mother with dementia describes how she and her brothers took turns in doing the practical things necessary to provide care.

> Between the three of us we were spelling each other off . . . you would get groceries, who would do this, who would do that?

A woman caring for her father with dementia described how her children also helped out.

> They [the children] take down his dinner for me. . . . Or go down and make his bed. . . . Just little things that they do to help.

A mother caring for a child with asthma and severe allergies had a friend who made and brought play dough and sterilized toys to her home.

> She brought play dough in, and she would make batches of play dough . . . she'd bring us books, or bring us a new batch of toys, because they all had to be sterilized before they came into T's room.

Other mothers of children with asthma or diabetes mentioned relatives who figured out what their child could have and brought meals, invited the family to a meal, or helped drive the child to appointments or school. Women caring for a relative with cancer appreciated the meals that neighbors or church members provided. A woman whose mother had cancer described how her son came to build a ramp for his grandmother and looked after the yard. Others mentioned help from a pharmacist who gave them free samples of medication or relatives who searched the Internet to locate less costly sources of medications. Mothers of infants mentioned help from their husbands or the infant's grandmother with housework and meals. Other examples from new mothers included caring for their dog, doing the grocery shopping, or caring for an older child while the parents visited their newborn in hospital.

One component of physical aid is respite care. Respite care provides a caregiver with temporary relief from her caregiving role. Women valued this form of support, as it gave them a much-needed break. Although we have included respite as a part of physical support, we recognize that there is an emotional component, as this assistance temporarily frees women from their responsibility as caregivers to pursue other interests that may have emotional benefits. Women described multiple examples of respite. Some illustrations follow.

> That is the most important, I think, that you have three days. Three days that I can go out in the morning and I don't have to worry. (**Caregiver of a relative with dementia**)

> I had a lot of help from child care services that the military had. They would take E [her son] even though he was three months old and colicky and screamed all the time. That was one of the few things that saved my sanity. (**Mother of a child with asthma and allergies**)

> When she got sicker and was in the hospital . . . and wanted to have someone there with her at all times, we took shifts. It was just invaluable. (**Woman caring for a relative with cancer**)

Information Support

We included information as a specific form of support, as women in all caregiving situations emphasized the high value of access to information. In some situations information was obtained from friends and family, but a consistent comment was the value of professionals such as doctors, nurses, and pharmacists who were willing to answer questions. The mother of a daughter with diabetes, who described her need for information in the form of "man in the street language" in a previous quote, was the sole parent for her daughter and initially relied on a source of information within her kin network.

Her father, the child's grandparent, was also diabetic, and he provided her with information on managing the disease. But, this information, provided by someone who was also a source of emotional support, differs from informational support from health professionals and was not suitable over time. A mother of an infant born prematurely described the informational support from professionals when she noted the importance of having her questions answered: "He [the physician] answers all of our questions."

Women caregivers offered many examples of information support. We include several additional illustrations. A woman caring for her mother with dementia appreciated information from her girlfriend about how to assist her mother.

> My girlfriend that's a nurse told me everything. I'd write all this down. She would tell me how to handle my mom, what to do.

A mother of a child with diabetes relied on a dietician for answers to questions about needed changes in her child's diet.

> The dietician has been the most helpful, like if I do need a question answered, I can phone her up, and she usually tries and gets the answer, and she phones back within a day or so.

The mother of a child with asthma had many questions that a medical intern was able to answer.

> His intern was fabulous. He gave me more information than anyone else in the hospital. He must have stayed about 20 minutes.

In summary, women in each of the caregiving situations described these three forms of support, and several noted that emotional support was the form of support most readily available to them. Although physical support and information support were important, women emphasized the value of being understood by someone who listened in a nonjudgmental way and was there for them. The nature of the relationships they had with others in their social networks provided the context for women's perceptions of support. In the following section, we discuss the dimensions of reciprocity and obligation in relationships within which women perceived support.

RELATIONSHIP DIMENSIONS OF RECIPROCITY AND OBLIGATION

Relationships with Family and Friends

Reciprocal exchange, or reciprocity, is believed to be an important dimension of social support among family and friends, as outlined in Chapter 1. In our research with family caregivers and mothers during a life transition, we explored the context in which reciprocity was present or absent, and the characteristics of reciprocity in the relationships of a caregiver with family and friends and the care recipient, as well as feelings about reciprocal exchanges during caregiving. Our research on reciprocity and social support included mothers of children and infants, including infants born prematurely, and women and men caring for a relative with dementia (Harrison & Neufeld, 1997; Harrison, Neufeld, & Kushner, 1995; Neufeld & Harrison, 1995, 1998).

We learned that there were different types of reciprocity. In relationships with kin and friends, the caregivers exhibited reciprocity, generalized reciprocity, and waived reciprocity. In relationships with a care recipient, caregivers exhibited generalized and waived reciprocity as well as a special form of reciprocity, constructed reciprocity. In the absence of reciprocity, they provided care in the context of obligation. Monitoring was a key process that facilitated reciprocity, particularly in the women's descriptions of their relationship with their relative (Neufeld & Harrison, 1995). This part of our research program did not address negotiated exchanges or the support provided by professionals, which is discussed in Chapter 5.

Women Caregivers

Reciprocity was an important dimension of women's supportive relationships with kin and friends, but was restricted in the relationships of some caregivers, thus limiting their access to support. Women were reluctant to seek support if they thought that they might be unable to reciprocate, as this could threaten the continuation of the relationship. One mother discussing child care commented,

> I feel better when I can reciprocate the help than [when it is] a one-sided affair.

Furthermore, a lack of reciprocity was perceived as an obstacle to the use of support. Although reciprocity was mentioned infrequently by mothers of full-term infants in their assessment of available support, mothers returning to work after an extended absence frequently discussed the importance of reciprocity. One mother asked neighbors to drive her children to community activities, but told the interviewer that she felt comfortable asking for assistance as she had provided the same help in the past.

> I haven't taken advantage of anybody; I had previously returned the favor ahead of time.

In relationships with friends and family members, women caring for an infant born prematurely or for a relative with dementia described reciprocity as a "give-and-take" that involved balancing the amount or kind of assistance exchanged. Usually give-and-take was manifested by distinct actions of support from friends and family or the caregiver, and occurred when a need for support was apparent. When caregiver gave support to family members or friends, their contribution of support allowed them to accept and use support from others when the need arose:

> You're not strong all the time. And when you are strong, you can give to the one who's not as strong at that time and it bounces back and forth. Then when you need some support, whether it's with your job or your child, you can take from the other person.

For these women, monitoring, reflecting, and making judgments about the presence of reciprocity occurred within the context of a specific time frame. The time span considered varied from an emphasis on the present and inclusion of the future to a broader scope that encompassed the past as well as the present. Some women noted that it was not always necessary to return the same kind of assistance as one received.

As reciprocity was considered essential to maintaining relationships. with members of their social network, the women constantly monitored the give-and-take. Their comments indicated that they kept a mental record of the balance between what they contributed and what they received. Participants described imbalances in their relationships, changes in the balance, and the perception that they owed much to others. As the following quote indicates, the general goal was to maintain an acceptable balance of give-and-take:

> It's not always fifty-fifty. Sometimes it's going to be ninety-ten. But you know it always comes out in the long run.

During caregiving, women caring for an infant born prematurely or a relative with dementia employed several cognitive strategies to maintain balanced reciprocity in their relationships with family and friends. Mothers of preterm infants stressed the future possibility of reciprocity and accepted assistance from people when they believed they could return the favor in the future. They anticipated that give-and-take between themselves and friends or kin would even out over time. Women caring for older adults maintained reciprocity by accepting assistance from friends and kin whom they had helped in the past and by helping those who had previously helped them. When the women were able to achieve reciprocity, the repeated give-and-take had several consequences. The reciprocal relationships became compatible and more committed, the women expressed improved self-esteem, and they found it easier to ask for assistance in their caregiving:

> There's a lot of satisfaction in knowing that you could do something for somebody else. The time may come when I need a lifeline.

A mother referred to reciprocity in the form of taking turns babysitting:

> I think if I clock a few hours looking after somebody else's kid, maybe I won't feel so bad asking them to look after mine.

However, an imbalance in reciprocity created problems that often resulted in fractured relationships:

> *Mother:* If someone is doing all the giving and somebody is doing all the taking, there is no relationship. That's like a parasite.
>
> *Interviewer:* If there wasn't give-and-take how would it affect a relationship?
>
> *Mother:* Over the long term? I don't think it would last that long. I think unless your life has been such that you're conditioned to give, and I mean there are people that are, I think a normal well-balanced person who recognizes their own needs, they're not going to stay in a relationship like that for long.

If the mothers felt there was no current or potential reciprocity between themselves and friends, they ended the relationships. Caregivers of older adults with dementia also ended relationships with friends when there was no reciprocity. However, in two instances, women caring for an older adult with dementia maintained relationships with friends who did not reciprocate. These women expressed a form of general reciprocity in which they contributed to friends without expecting a direct return. They gave support because they expected their friend to help someone else in turn ("pass it on") or simply because they valued giving to others. Women also tolerated a current lack of reciprocity with close family members by emphasizing the importance of family ties. They waived an expectation for immediate reciprocity and used an open-ended time period in which reciprocity could occur.

The type of reciprocity in a relationship had an impact on the feelings experienced by women caregivers. Women caring for an infant born prematurely or an adult with dementia and who engaged in reciprocal relationships with family and friends experienced positive feelings about themselves and their situation. However, they described mixed feelings, a combination of positive and negative feelings, about relationships in which they experienced a form of generalized or waived reciprocity.

Men Caregivers

Men caring for a relative with dementia valued reciprocity, but changes associated with caregiving led to issues in relationships with friends

Table 2.1

MEN'S RELATIONSHIPS WITH FAMILY AND FRIENDS: CHANGE, ISSUE, AND CONSEQUENCES FOR CAREGIVERS

Change	Issue	Consequences for Caregivers
Unable to reciprocate aid	Feelings of obligation	Reluctance to ask for help; preference for volunteered help; reliance on long-term reciprocal relationships
Unable to reciprocate in social activities	Loss of contact with friends	Feelings of anger, anxiety, and depression; substitution of social contact with agency, staff or community groups; formation of new relationships
Increased requirement	Unmet expectations	Relinquishment of expectations for family support; feelings of anger and difficulty in family relationships; acceptance of more limited forms of support for aid

and family that interfered with their ability to sustain reciprocity and support (see Table 2.1). These issues included a caregiver's feelings of obligation when unable to reciprocate aid, loss of contact with friends as the caregiver was unable to reciprocate socially, and unmet expectations as their need for family support increased. All of these issues affected the ability of a caregiver to access support, their feelings about caregiving and family relationships, and their opportunity for social interaction.

Many men who were caregivers were reluctant to request help because they felt obliged to return the favor and were unable to do so because of caregiving demands. Help that was volunteered was preferred:

> You feel obligated, and how do you even things out eventually? If they volunteer to help, that's fine.

Although these difficulties were expressed by most caregivers, one exception was a man who experienced consistent support and reciprocity in his relationships with family, friends, and neighbors. He described how his neighbors had looked after his house when he was away, and had arranged a 50th wedding anniversary party that included a visit to his home by his wife and other residents of the long-term care facility in which she lived. His relationships in the community were long-term and involved a lifetime of reciprocal interactions with family, friends, and neighbors.

A dominant theme for men caregivers was the withdrawal of friends from social activities. Caregivers were unable to accept spontaneous social invitations or reciprocate socially by inviting friends to their home. Also, as the care recipient's behavior changed, it became impossible for spousal caregivers to sustain their social role as a couple in relationships with friends. They found that it was difficult for friends to relate to the care recipient, and husbands missed the role their wives had formerly assumed in maintaining social contacts. As one man commented,

> The majority of people you had considered friends at one time just disappeared. As my wife became more demented it was difficult to find people to socialize with us.

Some men responded to the loss of friends with feelings of anger, anxiety, or depression. One caregiver, who felt very angry initially, later commented that things might have been better if he had been able to open up to his friends at the beginning. He wondered whether his friends would have understood if he had shared the problems of Alzheimer's disease when his wife could still have participated in social visits. Later, when the care recipient was admitted to long-term care, some friends again became more involved socially with the caregiver.

Several men, unable to maintain reciprocity in existing friendship relationships, replaced the social contact with other types of social inter-action. One caregiver visited a neighborhood restaurant several times a week. He made friends with the waitresses and the manager and said "It's like home." Another caregiver developed relationships with the staff in the long-term care facility where his wife lived. He volunteered assis-tance to many residents and their families and viewed the staff and the families of other residents as friends. For some men, participation in service clubs, community organizations, or support groups provided a new source of social interaction.

Two men formed new relationships with women while caring for their wives. These new relationships enabled them to continue social activities with friends as a couple. One man, a 77-year-old caregiver who had been married for over 50 years and whose wife was living in long-term care, described his new relationship as follows:

> She's the one I go out with, to a dance. To the family I gave her number because at times they can get me there.

The men described their new relationships as close and reciprocal, with exchanges of support:

> We share the cost of food, and she does the cooking.

As this quote illustrates, the support exchanged included assistance with daily activities.

For some men, there was an absence of reciprocity in family rela-tionships. They expected assistance from family members whom they had supported in the past. However, support was often not forthcoming from family members, whether they were immediate family or more dis-tant kin. In response, some caregivers accepted the status quo and relin-quished their expectations of aid by acknowledging that family members had other commitments. However, other men were angry at their family members' lack of participation in either visiting or assisting them or the care recipient. For some men, maintaining reciprocity with family members was difficult because their family members were separated geographically. When family members lived far away, more limited forms of support such as visits, telephone calls, and financial assistance were accepted as support and maintenance of reciprocity.

RELATIONSHIPS WITH THE CARE RECIPIENT

Women Caregivers

We explored reciprocity in the relationships of mothers with their prematurely born infants and the relationships of women caregivers with the relative with dementia for whom they provided care (Neufeld & Harrison, 1995). Because of the characteristics of the care recipient, the caregivers were unable to establish the same kind of reciprocal relationships as they did with others. Some of the caregivers recognized the distinction between reciprocity in the relationship with the care recipient and reciprocity in other relationships.

> In an ordinary relationship, the give and take are very important. We must remember though that there is something with illnesses which results in more take and less give.

Care recipients in this study were unable to communicate verbally and had other limitations that resulted in confused and ambiguous communication, which was a barrier to reciprocal relationships. As one mother commented,

> You don't expect give and take from a baby because they can't communicate.

Although reciprocity was important in the relationship with the care recipient, it took a different form. Most women developed a constructed reciprocity that was built through monitoring and reflecting.

Constructed Reciprocity Sustained by Monitoring and Reflecting

Caregivers shared detailed observations of the behavior and responses of the care recipient that they labeled as supportive actions. Particular attention was given to observations of nonverbal behaviors such as "You can see it in their [parents'] eyes" or "She's more alert now." One woman, who was caring for her mother, said, "I see recognition all the time in my mom's face, like when I go to pick her up." A mother commented, "He's young and a baby, the only way he can contribute is by his facial expression." Smiles were seen as the infant's positive feedback and a contribution to constructed reciprocity. The subprocess of observing was used to obtain evidence of meaningful interaction within the limited and confusing responses from the older adults with dementia and the immature premature infants.

A cognitive strategy used in conjunction with observation was to reduce expectations for a clear response from the care recipient and to label a responsive interaction as supportive. For example, participants accepted subtle and indistinct cues as responsive interaction. One mother of a small, ill, preterm infant, who used constructed reciprocity, recalled the effort involved when the infant was small:

> When she's [the baby] just lying there like a bump on the log, you think more about the interaction you're having with her. Whereas now you know you are having interaction with her.

This infant required extensive hospitalization. The mother described a progression from using subtle cues for interaction to relying on more distinct ones, which she associated with a close interaction with the child:

> She always held my finger when she was in the isolette and I stroked her . . . [now] if I come into her bedroom in the morning and she's chatting away to herself, as soon as she sees me, the biggest grin from ear to ear. It's just a very warm, close relationship.

A woman caring for her mother, who was now in a long-term care facility, described her mother's response to her physical care:

> When I rub her hand cream on or do anything like that, I usually find that she'll squeeze my hand or pat my hand or something like that.

As part of monitoring, mothers of premature infants and women caring for relatives with dementia used waiting and remembering in addition to observing. The mothers of preterm infants described waiting for the infants to mature and be more responsive. Caregivers of older adults described waiting for "good days," when the family member would remember them or recall a past experience:

> I thought that she was, like, totally, totally out of it, and yet at one time she piped up and said to me, "You made the apartment really nice." I realized that maybe she could think a little bit, and it probably comes and goes.

Remembering was described by mothers of preterm infants only in the sense that they recalled how the infant had behaved in recent weeks and noted the infant's increased responsiveness. Remembering past contributions from the care recipient was particularly important for caregivers of older persons. Often they were motivated by a desire to return what they had received in the past:

> I found myself sitting a lot of times thinking about the conversations we used to have. I value the memories.

Within the context of remembering and waiting, altering the time frame in which reciprocity was assessed was a common strategy. The caregivers of older adults considered and gave more weight to the contributions of the care recipient that they remembered from the distant past. However, if their main memory was of conflict or a lack of support in the history of the relationship, building a constructed reciprocity was impossible or very difficult. Extension of the time frame to the future meant anticipating intermittent signs of recognition or a response from the older adults. One woman caring for her mother-in-law, with whom she had previously had an excellent relationship and whom she greatly respected, said,

> There was so much giving before and I feel that all I'm giving now is certainly a part of this great big thing. But it doesn't, it's not the immediate day to day thing that's the give-and-take.

Mothers of preterm infants had a limited history to recall and consequently focused on the recent past. When building constructed reciprocity, they interpreted their infant's recent behavior as increasingly responsive. A mother whose infant was born at 28 weeks' gestational age and was hospitalized for 12 weeks commented in looking back over 18 months,

> It was really difficult. I got extremely tired, tired of him sometimes because he always seemed to be hanging on to me from one end to the other. But once he started smiling at us and acknowledging our existence and playing with us a little bit it got a lot easier.

Increasing responsiveness was interpreted as a hopeful sign that the baby would develop normally. The mothers of preterm infants emphasized the future and anticipated increasing reciprocity as their child matured.

When caregivers were able to construct reciprocity with their infants or older adults, they expressed contentment and satisfaction with themselves. One participant described satisfaction that her efforts to care for her mother-in-law were worthwhile.

> I take her somewhere [and] it seems to me, she really is looking around and she knows more about what's going on than she'll let on. I guess that gives me some satisfaction. It's worth doing this.

When mothers of preterm infants viewed the baby as responsive to their care, they felt rewarded:

> He'd [the baby] give you a real sappy look, and I didn't realize that that small of a baby was that expressive as far as their emotions. That's pretty rewarding.

Because of satisfaction and rewards experienced from a constructed reciprocity, both groups of caregivers described a closer relationship with the care recipient.

Waived Reciprocity

Three small subgroups of women did not develop a constructed reciprocity with the care recipient. These included those who waived an expectation of reciprocity, espoused general reciprocity in the form of altruism, or provided care on the basis of obligation.

A small subgroup of women waived an expectation for reciprocity because the care recipient's behavior was not perceived as intentional. Most of these women were mothers of preterm infants who indicated that the infant was not conscious of giving; therefore, they did not expect anything of the baby. They described feeling frustrated, depressed, bored, and burdened. By 6 to 8 months, however, when they perceived that the infants were able to respond to them through interactive play, the mothers shifted to building a constructed reciprocity. They then described feelings of satisfaction.

One woman caring for an older person said that a contribution could not be expected from her husband because of the nature of his illness. Although she indicated that she felt needed, she also described feeling guilty about admitting her husband to a long-term care facility, and tired and depressed when visiting. Unlike the mothers, she did not shift from waived reciprocity. Such a shift is unlikely in view of her husband's anticipated deterioration.

Generalized Reciprocity

The smallest category included only women who espoused an altruistic value commitment to continue to give without return. The women were all caring for an older adult. They described satisfaction but also expressed negative feelings about their situation. A woman who cared for her mother said she felt "drained." Her previous relationship with her mother, whom she described as controlling, was conflicted. Another woman, who was caring for her husband at home, described a positive relationship with him. She said that others viewed her as "someone with all her ducks in line," yet inwardly she felt desperate. Unlike the women who built a constructed reciprocity, women who espoused altruism had mixed feelings, feelings of satisfaction mixed with negative feelings such as sadness, anger, or desperation.

Obligation in the Absence of Reciprocity

In the absence of reciprocity, another subgroup of women referred to an obligation to care "because they're family" or because it was something they "should" do. Most women in this group were caring for older persons; two were mothers of preterm infants. Two examples of their views follow:

> She [the baby] didn't ask to be born; she's my responsibility.

> She's there and she's my mother, and I'll go as long as I can.

The mothers described their caregiving as very difficult and negatively overwhelming. They viewed the child as having a limited response to their caregiving, even at 12 months. In this subgroup, the caregivers of older persons described having to make sacrifices; feeling that they wanted to run away; being bitter or thinking, "What's the use?"; feeling that they "can't stand much more of it"; or feeling like they're always "on probation" because someone must know where they are. Two of these women also expressed positive feelings of satisfaction that the care recipient benefited from their care and, in one case, that they had previously had "a beautiful life together." It was not possible to determine whether the negative feelings described by the women were a consequence of their views of the caregiving relationship as an obligation or if they described caring as an obligation because of their negative feelings.

Men Caregivers

We also explored reciprocity in the relationships of men who were spouses and sons or grandsons and cared for a relative with dementia (Neufeld & Harrison, 1998). Similar to the women's descriptions, three variations in reciprocity in caregivers' relationship with the care recipient were identified: constructed reciprocity, waived reciprocity, and generalized reciprocity. The primary types of caregiving relationships evident among men caregivers were giving care on the basis of reciprocity and caring motivated by obligation in the absence of any form of reciprocity.

Those experiencing constructed or generalized reciprocity described positive feelings, whereas men identifying waived reciprocity described either positive or negative feelings. As with the women, when reciprocity was absent, the men described giving care based on obligation with either mixed or negative feelings.

Constructed Reciprocity

Similar to women caregivers in their experience of constructed reciprocity, men caregivers used observation and monitoring of their interaction with the care recipient, including attention to nonverbal behaviors. Subtle and indistinct nonverbal behaviors were described as a form of responsive interaction. The men who described constructed reciprocity with the care recipient were husbands who had a positive long-term relationship with their wives prior to the onset of dementia. Their focus was the unique characteristics of their wife as a person. The length of their marriages varied from 27 to 60 years, and they viewed the difficulties they faced through the lens of this relationship.

> The sadness of this disease has been counterbalanced by the 40-plus wonderful years we have enjoyed together.

Two men who were more articulate in describing their monitoring of nonverbal cues appeared to be influenced by their interaction with nursing staff in a long-term care facility. They observed nurses communicating with their family member and discussed the care recipient's responses with the staff. One man commented that he learned from watching nurses:

> The nurses say that even though she doesn't respond exactly, she looks more content when I am around. If I'm away for a week, when I get back, the biggest smiles . . . I think there's something still there that registers on some level. She will sometimes nod and shake her head and look at me and for a few seconds it will lock up and you can tell she's with you. But I talk to her anyway. A few nurses do the same thing.

Another man interpreted his wife's behavior when visiting her former home as interest and excitement, and this gave him a feeling of being connected with her:

> We brought her [his wife] in [to the house] and we just took her in all the rooms. She was looking, and something was there, because her head never stopped turning.

He also described other responses of his wife to his care.

> We [adult children and caregiver] get into the tea room . . . and get mom in the middle. It seems to do something for her because she seems content. There's something I'm sure gets through.

Although their statements include descriptions of several nonverbal behaviors, the men in the study reported primarily smiles, and their descriptions of observed behavior often lacked detail. Men who described constructed reciprocity expressed positive feelings about their relationship with the care recipient.

> I think there is a contact which does provide some source of energy to the person . . . it is good for me.

However, two caregivers who initially described a constructed reciprocity and positive feelings appeared to move throughout the period of the study from constructed reciprocity to obligation. As this change occurred, they expressed mixed feelings. One man gave brief descriptions of nonverbal behavior in early interviews, focusing on evidence of his wife's recognition of him. Later in the study, as he perceived fewer nonverbal cues, he described feeling obligated to provide care as a husband and expressed negative feelings. Another caregiver credited his wife of 27 years with helping him to achieve sobriety. In early interviews he portrayed the characteristics of constructed reciprocity by referring to nonverbal cues, which he interpreted as his wife's contribution to the relationship, and her continued influence in keeping him sober. By the end of the study, as he perceived that his wife recognized him less often, he made fewer references to her nonverbal cues, commented on his obligation to care for her, and increasingly expressed mixed feelings.

Waived Reciprocity

Although the men indicated that they valued reciprocity in relationships, some waived any expectation of immediate reciprocity because of the nature of the care recipient's illness. All of the men who waived reciprocity were husbands who had had a positive prior relationship with their wives and valued reciprocal exchanges, although they did not describe them within their current spousal relationship.

> My relationship with her now is as though she was a child and I was looking after her. You have to do what you have to do.

These caregivers described their caregiving in a factual manner and indicated that the care recipients could contribute little because of their impairment. Caregivers who waived reciprocity were content to contribute to the care recipient on the basis of the care recipient's current needs. They gave no descriptions of the care recipients' non-verbal behaviors or response either to them or to health professionals. In addition, they did not suggest that their care arose from the desire to return past contributions of the care recipient. Two of these caregivers noted that the care recipient no longer recognized them. Some of the men who gave care in the context of waived reciprocity expressed positive feelings, whereas others described negative feelings about caregiving.

Generalized Reciprocity

A grandson in this study expressed a high personal commitment to altruistic values and the view that the assistance offered would not be returned by the recipient but would be passed on in a larger sense of community. He valued the role of caregiving for his grandmother as a model for his children in understanding the importance of contributing to others. He experienced satisfaction in his caregiving role:

> She provides what I like to see, what I would try to provide for my children, that there are going to be responsibilities, not so much to society, but in a larger sense. She [my grandmother] took care of her grandmother, her mother, and her sister.

In this way, he attached importance to the contribution that his grandmother and others of her generation had made to society and to family members. He also saw his caregiving as the expression of a general altruistic value of contribution to a larger good, a value he wanted to communicate to his children. Although his grandmother, whom he had not known well as a child, no longer recognized him, he described his visits with her in positive terms. His descriptions include no reference to his grandmother's nonverbal responses or behaviors.

Obligation in the Absence of Reciprocity

Most of the men described giving care based on obligation without any form of reciprocity. This group of caregivers included those who were caring for a parent or parent-in-law, a sibling, and several who were the husband or partner of the care recipient. The obligation to care for a family member was based on a feeling that they "ought" to care for their family member because of their relationship. One man, caring for his brother, saw himself as the family member responsible to protect and rescue his siblings. He was one of 12 children who had lost their mother early in life and were later abandoned by their father. This group of caregivers frequently used the word "obligation"; for example,

> I feel obligated. It's my responsibility. I've been having obligations since I was a kid. They [siblings] all depended on me. I still feel an obligation to go over and visit with her [mother]. We've got to look after our parents. We can't just put them in homes and expect strangers to look after them.

Most men whose caring was motivated by obligation had experienced a positive relationship with the care recipient prior to his or her illness, although some described their previous relationship as ambivalent or conflicted. Many of the men who gave care as a result of obligation described feeling burdened, stressed, angry, alone, and frustrated with their situation:

> I do get really frustrated.... You want to bang your head against the wall.

A few expressed mixed feelings about caregiving, simultaneously talking about their frustration with their situation and their satisfaction that the care recipient had good care. In Figure 2.1 we summarize the findings concerning reciprocity and obligation in the caregiving relationships of men.

Two factors influenced men's perspectives. As indicated in Figure 2.1, the first was the relationship with the care recipient prior to caregiving. Both the quality of the relationship (positive, negative, reciprocal, or nonreciprocal) and the type of family role influenced the present interaction. Those caring by constructed, waived, or generalized reciprocity described a positive, reciprocal prior relationship with the care recipient and a motivation to care based either on the unique characteristics of the individual care recipient (constructed reciprocity) or on a belief in reciprocity as a social norm. The motivation for men caring by obligation was the belief that caring was required by their family role as a husband, brother, or son. In this group the quality of the prior relationship varied; most described positive, reciprocal prior relationships, but some characterized their prior relationship as ambivalent or conflicted.

The second influencing factor was exposure to the example of nurses, who assisted some of the men by describing nonverbal cues to help the

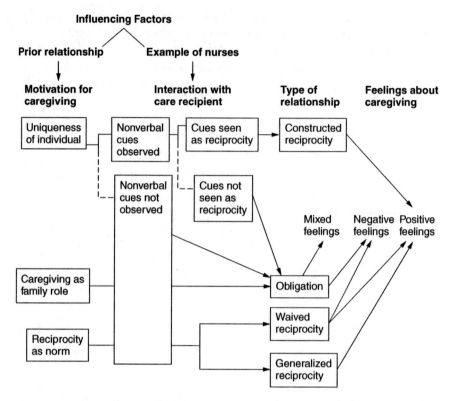

Figure 2.1. Reciprocity and obligation in the relationship with the care recipient.

men interpret these cues as feedback from the care recipient. In this way nurses in long-term care assisted caregivers in their interaction and enabled them to establish a relationship of constructed reciprocity with their wives.

The men's motivation for caregiving influenced their interpretations of the care recipient's behavior. If they focused primarily on the unique characteristics of the individual care recipient, they described nonverbal behavior and interpreted this as a form of reciprocal exchange, which we have identified as constructed reciprocity. On the other hand, when their motivation to care was a belief that their family role (e.g., of spouse or sibling) required caregiving, there was no description of the subtle behavioral cues given by the care recipient or discussion of current reciprocity in the relationship. These caregivers performed their caregiving role based on obligation. When caregivers believed that the norm of reciprocity should be suspended under certain conditions or could be met through contributions to a third party, they described either waived or generalized reciprocity in the caregiving relationship but did not describe observations of nonverbal cues given by the care recipient.

The perception of reciprocity in the caregiving relationship was related to the men's feelings about their caregiving. Those who established constructed reciprocity in the relationship with the care recipient or who portrayed generalized reciprocity had positive feelings. Men who perceived the caregiving relationship in terms of obligation described either negative or mixed feelings; men who waived expectations of reciprocity had either positive or negative feelings.

A change occurring for two caregivers over the course of the study is portrayed by the series of dotted lines in Figure 2.1. These men failed to sustain a focus on the unique characteristics of their wives and described fewer interpretations of nonverbal behavioral cues over the duration of the study. Their initial descriptions were characteristic of constructed reciprocity and associated with positive feelings. However, by the end of the study they no longer mentioned the nonverbal responses of their wives, referring instead to obligation as a caregiver, and expressed negative feelings.

DISCUSSION

Reciprocity was present and important in relationships with family and friends for both women and men caregivers and has been identified by other researchers (Hayes, 2006). These findings support the theoretical perspective of social exchange theory (Cook & Rice, 2003; Homans, 1961) and the importance of reciprocal exchanges in social interactions with family and friends (Molm, Quist, & Wisely, 1994). Implicit in this perspective is the recognition that reciprocal exchanges are necessary for the continuation of social relationships (Langford, Bowsher, Maloney, & Lillis, 1997). However, the type of support exchanged does not need to be similar. For example Lowenstein and colleagues (Lowenstein, Katz, & Gur-Yaish, 2007) reported reciprocal exchanges between adult children and their parents, with adult children providing instrumental support, their parents providing financial support, and both exchanging emotional support. Reciprocal exchanges can be influenced by factors such as decreased health in one member of the dyad with diminished ability for reciprocity (Lyons,

Sayer, Archbold, Hornbrook, & Stewart, 2007). Decreased reciprocity may increase the cost of caregiving and affect the stability of the relationship or change the nature of the caregiving relationship to one of obligation.

Reciprocity in the exchange of support may influence mood. In related research on the daily exchange of support within intimate relationships, reciprocity between partners was associated with higher levels of positive mood and lower levels of negative mood, whereas receiving support without reciprocation was associated with increased negative mood (Gleason, Iida, Bolger, & Shrout, 2003). Although this study did not address a caregiving situation or an extended time frame, the findings are congruent with the descriptions of participants in our research.

Among participants in our research, nonreciprocal relationships with friends were often terminated, whereas expectations for reciprocity were sometimes waived with family members. Termination of nonreciprocal relationships may conserve resources for other relationships and caregiving but could also reduce the number of available sources of support. Alternatively, termination of nonreciprocal relationships could also enable caregivers to receive support from more valued sources. Caregivers who maintained nonreciprocal relationships demonstrated what we called generalized reciprocity, that is, giving without an expectation of personal benefit, which has also been termed third-party reciprocity or altruism (Antonucci & Akiyama, 1987; Avioli, 1989; Nye, 1979). A study of family caregiving in Taiwan, in which daughters-in-law did most of the family caregiving, further confirms the role of generalized reciprocity (Hsu & Shyu, 2003). Among these caregivers, caregiving was seen as an investment in rewards that will come in the future and will be repaid by someone other than the elder for whom they care. A finding from research on couples' daily exchange of support also affirms the potential benefit for caregivers of engaging in generalized reciprocity as giving of support without receiving assistance was associated with a decrease in negative mood whereas receiving support without reciprocation was associated with an increase in negative mood (Gleason, Iida, Bolger, & Shrout, 2003).

In their relationships with care recipients, men and women demonstrated similar forms of reciprocity and, in the absence of reciprocity, described giving care by obligation. When care recipients had limited ability to reciprocate, many women interacted with them through a constructed reciprocity. These women expressed positive feelings toward the care recipient and less distress in their caregiving role than women who viewed themselves as caring through obligation did. Men exhibited similar forms of reciprocity, including constructed reciprocity, but there were some differences. Fewer men than women employed constructed reciprocity, and two of the men appeared over the course of the study to be in a process of transition from constructed reciprocity to a perception of obligation. In an Australian study of caregiver burden among men and women caring for someone with disability, illness, or frailty due to aging, reciprocity was found to decrease caregiver burden (Reid, Moss, & Hyman, 2005). Of interest to us is the suggestion by Reid and colleagues that the contribution of the care recipient in the form of expressions of gratitude to the caregiver and warmth in the relationship may have potential to diminish caregiver burden. In relationships with relatives with advanced dementia or prematurity, expressions of gratitude to the caregiver may not be possible, but in our research, caregivers' descriptions of constructed reciprocity accompanied by positive feelings may represent their construction of an alternate form of nonverbal feedback from the care recipient that is congruent with this interpretation.

There is no obvious explanation as to why women were more likely than men to describe constructed reciprocity with the care recipient, although men who engaged in constructed reciprocity were much less explicit than the women were in describing the nonverbal cues that were interpreted as a component of their interaction. Men described primarily smiles of the care recipient but not other nonverbal behaviors. One possible explanation may be women's greater facility and men's limited skill in decoding nonverbal cues (Hall, 1984). Other researchers found in a study of couple relationships, not necessarily caregiving relationships, that women were more attentive to the specific content in supportive interactions than were men, who focused more on the overall nature of the message and their perception of the couple relationship (Carels & Baucom, 1999). Carels and Baucom suggest that men filter information on interactions in their relationships differently than women, but this idea needs further testing.

In our findings, each man who described constructed reciprocity also had a positive long-term relationship with his wife who was the care recipient. This is congruent with other findings (Wright, 1993), which have indicated that in spite of their spouse's dementia, caregivers who experienced marital happiness in the past were able to value the uniqueness of their spouse and talk of a loving relationship in the present. Others (Bleiszner & Shifflett, 1990) have found that over time, spouses who lost communication with a care recipient spouse redefined their relationship, with an emphasis on loyalty to the care recipient rather than interaction in the relationship. This might be similar to the process involving the men who moved from constructed reciprocity to caring by obligation.

Our findings on perception of the meaning of support and the types of supportive interactions were also congruent with findings of other research. For women caregivers in our research, the meaning of support involved having someone who would share their experience, be a sounding board, and offer them objective feedback. This view of the meaning of support is similar to findings of a phenomenological study of the meaning of support among family caregivers caring for a senior relative in Sweden (Stoltz, Willman, & Uden, 2006) in which family caregivers referred to support as experiencing togetherness with others in sharing the responsibility and hardship.

Similarly, the descriptions in our research of types of supportive interactions reflect components of support similar to the findings of other researchers: emotional support, physical support, and informational support. In a concept analysis of social support, others have identified similar components of social support, including emotional support, instrumental support, informational support, and appraisal support (Langford, et al., 1997). Appraisal support refers to information that is relevant to self-evaluation rather than problem solving; some (Kahn & Antonucci, 1980) have used the term *affirmational support* to describe statements that affirm acts of another. This latter meaning is similar to women caregivers' descriptions of feedback from others about their caregiving role, which we have included as appraisal support and a component of emotional support. Similar to our findings, some other researchers (Cohen, 2004; Dunkel-Schetter, Folkman, & Lazarus, 1987) have also suggested emotional, instrumental, and informational support as categories for types of support.

In summary, our findings affirm the meaning and importance of social support for women and men caregivers and the influence of reciprocity and obligation in the relationships of family caregivers for their experience of support. In our findings, variations in caregivers' experience of support and reciprocity as they interact with others in their social network are associated with differing emotional states. Identification of the presence or absence of support and the type of reciprocity between a caregiver and members of their social network can facilitate a professional's understanding of caregivers' perceptions and suggest ways that the professional can enhance a caregiver's ability to foster supportive interactions.

NOTE

The data reported in this chapter were drawn from the studies of women and men caregivers that were reported in Harrison & Neufeld (1997); Harrison, Neufeld, & Kushner (1995); Neufeld & Harrison (1995, 1998); and Neufeld, Harrison, Hughes, & Stewart (2007).

REFERENCES

Antonucci, T. C., & Akiyama, H. (1987). Social networks in adult life and a preliminary examination of the convoy model. *Journal of Gerontology, 42,* 519–527.

Avioli, P. S. (1989). The social support functions of siblings in later life. *American Behavioral Scientist, 33*(1), 45–57.

Bleiszner, R., & Shifflett, P. (1990). The effects of Alzheimer's disease on close relationships between patients and caregivers. *Family Relations, 39,* 57–62.

Carels, R. A., & Baucom, D. H. (1999). Support in marriage: Factors associated with online perceptions of support helpfulness. *Journal of Family Psychology, 13,* 131–144.

Cohen, S. (2004). Social relationships and health. *American Psychologist, 59*(8), 676–684.

Cook, K. S., & Rice, E. (2003). Social exchange theory. In J. Delamater (Ed.), *Handbook of social psychology* (pp. 53–76). New York: Kluwer Academic/Plenum.

Dunkel-Schetter, C., Blasband, D. E., Feinstein, L. G., & Herbert, T. B. (1992). Elements of supportive interactions: When are attempts to help effective? In S. Spacapan & S. Oskamp (Eds.), *Helping and being helped: Naturalistic studies* (pp. 83–114). Newbury Park, CA: Sage.

Dunkel-Schetter, C. C., Folkman, S., & Lazarus, R. S. (1987). Correlates of social support receipt. *Journal of Personality and Social Psychology, 53,* 71–80.

Funch, D. P., Marshall, J. R., & Gebhardt, G. P. (1986). Assessment of a short scale to measure social support. *Social Science & Medicine, 23*(3), 337–344.

Gleason, M. E. J., Iida, M., Bolger, N., & Shrout, P. E. (2003). Daily supportive equity in close relationships. *Personality and Social Psychology Bulletin, 29,* 1036–1045.

Hall, J. (1984). *Nonverbal sex differences: Communication accuracy and expertise.* Baltimore: Johns Hopkins University Press.

Harrison, M. J., & Neufeld, A. (1997). Women's experiences of barriers to support while caregiving. *Health Care for Women International, 18,* 591–602.

Harrison, M. J., Neufeld, A., & Kushner, K. (1995). Women in transition: Access and barriers to support. *Journal of Advanced Nursing, 21,* 858–864.

Hayes, P. (2006). Home is where their health is: Rethinking perspectives of informal and formal care by older rural Appalachian women who live alone. *Qualitative Health Research, 16*(2), 282–297.

Homans, G. C. (1961). *Social behavior and its elementary forms.* New York: Harcourt, Brace and World.

Hsu, H-C., & Shyu, Y-I. L. (2003). Implicit exchanges in family caregiving for frail elders in Taiwan. *Qualitative Health Research, 13,* 1078–1093.

Kahn, T. L., & Antonucci, T. C. (1980). Convoys over the life course: Attachment, roles, and social support. *Life Span Development and Behavior, 3,* 269–276.

Langford, C. P. H., Bowsher, J., Maloney, J. P., & Lillis, P. P. (1997). Social support: A conceptual analysis. *Journal of Advanced Nursing, 25*(1), 95–100.

Lowenstein, A., Katz, R., & Gur-Yaish, N. (2007). Reciprocity in parent-child exchange and life satisfaction among the elderly: A cross-national perspective. *Journal of Social Issues, 63*(4), 865–883.

Lyons, K. S., Sayer, A. G., Archbold, P. G., Hornbrook, M. C., & Stewart, B. J. (2007). The enduring and contextual effects of physical health and depression on care-dyad mutuality. *Research in Nursing & Health, 30*, 84–98.

Molm, L. D., Quist, T. M., & Wisely, P. A. (1994). Imbalanced structures, unfair strategies: Power and justice in social exchange. *American Sociological Review, 59*, 98–121.

Neufeld, A., & Harrison, M. J. (1995). Reciprocity and social support in caregivers' relationships: Variations and consequences. *Qualitative Health Research, 5*, 348–365.

Neufeld, A., & Harrison, M. J. (1998). Men as caregivers: Reciprocal relationships or obligation? *Journal of Advanced Nursing, 28*, 959–968.

Neufeld, A., Harrison, M. J., Hughes, K., & Stewart, M. (2007). Nonsupportive interactions in the experience of women family caregivers. *Health and Social Care in the Community, 15*(6), 530–541.

Nye, F. (1979). Choice, exchange, and the family. In W. R. Burr, R. Hill, F. I. Nye, & I. L. Reiss (Eds.), *Contemporary theories about the family* (Vol. 2, pp. 1–41). New York: Macmillan.

Reid, C. E., Moss, S., & Hyman, G. (2005). Caregiver reciprocity: The effects of reciprocity, carer self-esteem and motivation on the experience of caregiver burden. *Australian Journal of Psychology, 57*, 186–196.

Stoltz, P., Willman, A., & Uden, G. (2006). The meaning of support as narrated by family carers who care for a senior relative at home. *Qualitative Health Research, 16*(5), 594–610.

Wright, L. K. (1993). *Alzheimer's disease and marriage.* Newbury Park, CA: Sage.

3

Nonsupportive Interactions in Varied Caregiving Situations

In addition to relationship dimensions such as reciprocity or obligation, family caregivers in our research on social support held specific expectations that guided their appraisal and evaluation of the content of interactions as either supportive or nonsupportive. As caregivers monitored and reflected on their interactions with members of their social network, they evaluated some of those interactions as nonsupportive. For example, as indicated in Chapter 2, mothers experiencing a transition, such as the birth of their first child or returning to work after an extended absence, described support as having someone to talk to, someone who listened and allowed them to explore ideas. Listeners were supportive when they were reliable and available, allowed the woman to make her own choices, and offered their assistance. Implicit in these descriptions were expectations of others that, when fulfilled, were appraised as supportive or, when unfulfilled, were considered nonsupportive. As confirmed in a study of women caregivers, these expectations were rooted in caregivers' personal beliefs and values, as well as their caregiving context and social situation.

Although research has often viewed social support as unconditionally positive, there is evidence that negative interactions, such as conflict and dissatisfaction with support, are present in caregivers' relationships (Carpentier & Ducharme, 2005; Pesiah, Brodaty, & Quadrio, 2006; Ray, 2002; Sullivan-Bolyai, Deatrick, Gruppuso, Tamborlane, & Grey, 2003; Wuest, Ericson, Stern, & Irwin, 2001). Nonsupportive interactions can be embedded within supportive relationships (Pesiah et al., 2006; Wuest et al., 2001) and have an influence on caregivers' psychological health (Cohen, 2004).

In this chapter we describe nonsupportive interactions and the relationship between expectations of support and the experience of nonsupport. We outline the forms of nonsupportive interactions and related conditions that were identified in our studies. These findings are then discussed in relation to other research in caregiving situations and relevant theoretical concepts in social exchange and ecological theory.

EXPECTATIONS AND PERCEPTIONS OF NONSUPPORTIVE INTERACTIONS

In a study of mothers experiencing the transition of the birth of their first child or of returning to work after an extended absence, women described nonsupportive interactions as unhelpful comments or actions from someone who was supportive in other ways. Support and nonsupport were seen to coexist in the same relationships. For example, one mother described leaving her infant with her mother-in-law, who was willing to babysit. When she returned, she found that her mother-in-law had cut the infant's hair without discussing this with her, so she decided not to ask for further assistance from her mother-in-law. In another example, a mother stopped accepting her grandmother's offers of babysitting because of the nonsupportive comments that she received on her mothering skills:

> You don't feed the boy enough. He's starving, no wonder he's crying.

> Cut the feet out of his sleeper. Are you trying to strangle him?

Both women expected that the assistance they received from family members would support them in their role as a mother in addition to receiving assistance in child care.

Mothers returning to work also expressed dissatisfaction with the support they received from their families. They were often the recipients of nonsupportive comments or acts when their work outside the home made it difficult for them to carry out responsibilities at home. One woman reported that her husband and three children said she was "doing too much." She recognized that this message was nonsupportive and not an expression of concern for her:

> I'm doing what I can, and I feel OK about it, like, leave me. As much as they [her husband and children] want to complain, they also realize that the solution is not easy.

Possible solutions to her work overload included quitting work or having her family provide help in the house. Because the family members did not respond to their observation of her "doing too much" with any increase in their contributions to household management, the woman received the unspoken message that she should reconsider working outside the home. Subsequently, she quit her job and returned to work only when she found a position with fewer demands on her.

Descriptions of Nonsupportive Interactions in Studies of Family Caregiving

Descriptions of nonsupportive interactions recurred in our studies of family caregivers. In a study of women caring for a relative with dementia, women caregivers described nonsupportive interactions with family and friends that included disparaging comments belittling the caregiver and criticism of her decisions related to the care recipient. For example, one woman felt belittled and unable to express her views when a friend in the church dismissed her concern that support for the poor was inadequate but that elected members of the government were receiving pay increases. This caregiver experienced severe poverty and heavy demands, arising from her responsibility to care for her two young grandchildren in addition to her husband, who had dementia:

> I was pretty uptight over something that had happened with Social Services. I brought up the subject . . . "Listen, people are not getting enough financial assistance." Now this lady also has someone who is within the government, an MP [Member of Parliament], and I had said something to her . . . about MPs getting the big raise and the poor not getting anything . . . I was just shut right out.

Several caregivers experienced criticism from family members. One woman recounted that her family made joking remarks, such as "Can't you do that?" or "Are you losing it?" Another example is a woman whose brother blamed her for withdrawing from the family and was critical of her husband, who had dementia:

> I said, ". . . the doctor suspects he has Alzheimer's, and I just ask that you let the kids know." I went away in tears because my brother just went up one side of my spine and down the other, just tearing into me [about] withdrawing from the family.

Women caring for a relative with dementia also described conflict between themselves and others in their appraisal of the care recipient's health status. For example, family and friends did not believe a caregiver's description of her relative's need for assistance. A woman felt that her husband's family denied his illness, blamed her husband for his emerging negative behavior, and withdrew from social contact—despite her efforts to interpret his behavior as a reflection of his dementia. As a result of this dissonance, relationships that had been close were disrupted:

> I guess it's denial . . . there's just no help there. They don't want to have Dave [a pseudonym] around. Boy, that hurts. He was the uncle that was supposedly the special one, he was the one that did everything for all the nieces and nephews. They accepted all his help.

A granddaughter caring for her grandmother was frustrated with her mother's approach to helping her. She wanted her mother to assist with grocery shopping. However, her mother chose to provide social interaction for the grandmother.

> What she'll do is she'll do things that she likes doing. Like my mom likes bingo, so she takes my grandmother to bingo, because she likes doing that. But it probably would not occur to her to take her grocery shopping.

Other examples included a visitor from the church who took the care recipient out for such a short time that it provided no respite for the caregiver and a friend who assisted the caregiver with grocery shopping in a way that did not meet her needs.

> But if he [the friend] goes with me for groceries, he keeps coming up to me every 5 minutes, "What do you need now?" He's always hurrying me because everything has to be done in a very business-like manner.

These examples illustrate a caregiver's unfulfilled expectations for support. These unfulfilled expectations were particularly disappointing when they took the form of offers or promises of assistance that were not fulfilled. One woman described her disappointment when promised support did not materialize.

> So many times people have said, "Oh I'm going to have tea with you one of these days." Or "So-and-so and I are going to come and visit you, and my husband will stay with your husband, and you and I will go shopping." But it never happens. So you lose faith in people after awhile.

Disappointment in situations such as this was especially acute because the women's expectations were grounded in explicit offers of assistance.

Support and nonsupport often coexisted in relationships. One caregiver who received assistance from her son and daughter-in-law nevertheless found that they were critical of the way she handled her affairs and expected her to be more dependent than she wished—for example, advising them each time she went out.

> They expect you . . . to be dependent . . . If he [the son] phones me and says "I tried to phone you two or three times and you weren't home, now where were you?" Now do I have to report in? "Yes, you should, I worry about you."

Sometimes support and nonsupport alternated over time in a relationship. A brother and sister-in-law of one caregiver withdrew their support, but when they eventually accepted her husband's diagnosis of dementia, they established some contact and provided support.

> My brother and his wife came over . . . on the day that I had gotten the phone call . . . that I had to have a [breast] biopsy. Ethel then said, "If you want John to stay with us or we can help you, we'd be glad to." . . . maybe they would then see what the score was . . . they were good to him.

Forms of Nonsupportive Interactions

Although descriptions of nonsupportive interactions were present in several of our earlier studies, we specifically examined the types of nonsupportive interactions experienced in a study of women caregivers in four caregiving situations: mothers caring for an infant born prematurely or for a child with asthma or diabetes, and women caring for an adult with cancer or dementia. The nonsupportive interactions caregivers experienced took three major forms: negative actions that undermined their credibility as caregivers, interactions in which the intended aid was ineffective, or interactions in which expected support was absent. Each of these forms of nonsupportive interactions included a range of specific subcategories. Caregivers' perceptions indicated that the forms of nonsupportive interactions were common across all caregiving situations.

Interactions classified as negative refer to actions the women perceived as offensive and undermining. Negative interactions included discounting in the form of minimizing caregivers' concerns, not understanding their intent, or not believing their stories. Other negative behaviors included blaming or criticizing the caregiving, refusing to give the support the caregiver requested, intimidating the caregiver, or expressing disrespect for the woman as a person.

Ineffective interactions involved actions intended to be helpful but perceived as not providing the assistance needed. Ineffective actions included inadequate provision of information, inappropriate advice, or other inadequate or inappropriate gestures of support.

Absence of expected or desired support occurred when someone who was expected to be supportive failed to recognize the woman's need or did not give assistance. This form of nonsupportive interaction included not recognizing a caregiver's need for help; being intimidated by the situation; being in conflict with the caregiver; not providing the help that a caregiver expected, including restricted or nonexistent service; lack of connection to friends and family; and making promises of help that were not realized.

These nonsupportive interactions are illustrated in Table 3.1. In the table, we present a summary of the forms of nonsupportive interactions, the subcategories of each form, and illustrative comments from family caregivers. In addition to the illustrations presented in the table, we provide further examples of ineffective forms of support to illustrate the perspectives of caregivers in more detail.

For several reasons, women appraised as nonsupportive offers of help that were not what they needed. They could not rely on the assistance that was offered, the assistance was unpredictable and inconsistent, or the help was offered by people who lacked the skills needed to provide care. Examples included offers to do the laundry by someone who ruined the clothes, or offers to babysit a child with diabetes from people who could not give the necessary injections. When members of their social network made inquiries for information but did not offer to help, women

Table 3.1

CATEGORIES OF NONSUPPORTIVE INTERACTIONS WITH EXAMPLES

Caregiver Group and Situation		A = Woman Caring for Relative with Dementia C = Mother of Child with Diabetes or Asthma
		B = Woman Caring for Relative/Friend with Cancer D = Mother of Infant Born Prematurely
Category	Subcategory	Example Quotation by Caregiving Situation
1.0 Negative	1.1 Discounting; minimizing	A: He [CG's brother] consistently tells me that I'm making a big thing out of nothing, because, you know, "They're fine" [CG's parents] when he talks to them on the phone.
		C: Even with professional people, like pharmacists, they'll say, oh, well, she'll grow out of it.
	Not understanding	C: It's like my mother saying, oh, give him [CG's son with asthma] a little chocolate, it won't hurt him. No, it'll just kill him, you know, he cannot have chocolate, period. Most people are not willing to take that extra step to understand.
		D: People don't, don't understand because they just don't get it! Especially if you're dealing with a sick one [premature infant], if you have two perfectly healthy kids it's easy to a certain extent, but if you're running a household and you're managing and you're taking care of everything else that goes along with life, it's hard, and people don't get it.
	Disbelieving	A: And so, she [a general practitioner] decided that that my mom was still charmingly gaudy, but I was such a bag that she gave [my mom] the geriatric assessment [to diagnose cognitive impairment] just to keep me out of her waiting room.
		C: And, over the years, she's [the child's grandmother] gotten a lot better. . . . But she was in major denial, for the worst part of it. She just could not accept that that could be like that.
	1.2 Blaming	B: The day of D.'s [relative with cancer] biopsy, the admitting nurse was, like, mad at me, and like, "How could you, as a mother?"

(Continued)

Table 3.1

CATEGORIES OF NONSUPPORTIVE INTERACTIONS WITH EXAMPLES *(continued)*

Caregiver Group and Situation		A = Woman Caring for Relative with Dementia B = Woman Caring for Relative/Friend with Cancer	C = Mother of Child with Diabetes or Asthma D = Mother of Infant Born Prematurely
Category	Subcategory	Example Quotation by Caregiving Situation	
		C: It's [child's diabetes] not my fault. I didn't do something in pregnancy that caused this. Why are you blaming us for a fluke of nature on a chromosome? Why are you blaming us for this, and why are you denying us this help?	
	1.3 Refusing to give support	A: She [relative with dementia] was acting that way, and I said, oh, you know, I think she's got a urine infection, please check her out. And they [the nurses] just wouldn't. They absolutely refused.	
	1.4 Intimidating	C: I went . . . to my worker, and I said, "We need a new monitor." She said, "Oh, we don't pay for that." They don't pay for the monitors anymore. They pay for one every five years. And they don't pay for her lancets.	
		A: I get kinda of tongue-tied when I have to talk to her. . . . I think maybe I'm not I'm not explaining it properly, simply for the fact that I feel—and, you know, "intimidated" might not be the right word, but along those lines, you know.	
		D: I would have breast fed if I had a choice, and I still find, even now, some nurses, you know, really, really trying to talk me into it. And, and it's like, you know what, I've made my decision . . . I have my reasoning . . . You can leave me alone now. . . . So many of them [the nurses] are so adamant about it. They really try to push you, and then some try to push a little too much.	
	1.5 Disrespecting	C: I just really was sick of it, because I got the impression, like, from everybody, that their whole attitude was that I didn't know anything; I was just this, you know, loser who wasn't managing well.	
		D: You may be a nurse, and you maybe have taken five years [of school], but I'm not stupid either. You know, I may have maybe a different [out]look on it. I'm tired of people walking all over me.	

Table 3.1

CATEGORIES OF NONSUPPORTIVE INTERACTIONS WITH EXAMPLES *(continued)*

Caregiver Group and Situation		A = Woman Caring for Relative with Dementia B = Woman Caring for Relative/Friend with Cancer	C = Mother of Child with Diabetes or Asthma D = Mother of Infant Born Prematurely
Category	**Subcategory**	**Example Quotation by Caregiving Situation**	
2.0 Ineffective	2.1 Inadequate information	B: We would come out of there [the doctor's office], my mom, my dad, and I. And we'd have three different interpretations of what the doctor or nurse had said. And we'd kind of battle it out and come to some understanding.	
		C: You'll always run into the well-meaning people again; they try and pave the way for you, and they don't necessarily give the right information.	
	2.2 Inappropriate advice	B: The doctor shouldn't just give you a blank statement like that, "Don't worry," because if you know something's going on with your family member, and they're still doing more tests or whatever, it's very hard not to worry, and just telling you not to worry is not going to be very helpful at all.	
		D: People would, um, trivialize it [caring for a premature infant], by saying things like, well if you're so tired and you're [not] getting any sleep, quit breast feeding and let them cry. Okay, that was not the solution that I wanted to hear, you know, and it absolutely bugged [me].	
	2.3 Other inadequate/ inappropriate gestures of dupport	A: And so, it's an offer [of support], and it's like, okay, thank you, but . . . but it's not exactly what I need, you know.	
		B: I have a lot of people doing verbal support, which means absolutely nothing to you when you're frustrated and running around and worrying.	
3.0 Absence of expected support	3.1 Need is unrecognized	A: I found that really frustrating, to go through the system when you . . . when you have to justify everything that you need, when you have to, like, beg and plead and whine for things that somebody should just, just have given you.	

(Continued)

Table 3.1

CATEGORIES OF NONSUPPORTIVE INTERACTIONS WITH EXAMPLES *(continued)*

Caregiver Group and Situation		A = Woman Caring for Relative with Dementia B = Woman Caring for Relative/Friend with Cancer	C = Mother of Child with Diabetes or Asthma D = Mother of Infant Born Prematurely
Category	Subcategory	Example Quotation by Caregiving Situation	
		B: When you want help, and they're not there to help you. When you want the mental help, and they're not there to help you. Those are the very cold nonsupporters.	
	3.2 Helper is intimidated	A. Nobody even wants to suggest helping. I think they're afraid of the responsibility. C: A lot of people are scared to offer to [do] that [to watch her child]. Because usually that means needles, and a lot of people are scared of needles.	
	3.3 No potential for support, as a result of conflict	A: I've done nothing to hurt them. . . . To get treated like this, I don't like it. . . . His brother hasn't spoken to me since the day after he died, the day of his death when I phoned to let him know. I haven't heard from him. D: I think it was just more personal conflicts around; for example, P.'s parents would come from W, which is an hour away. And, but they didn't want to intrude, so they would only stay a couple of minutes. That was annoying in itself. . . . They're really, they're really anxious to get out of there.	
	3.4 Help is not available		
	Service is restricted or nonexistent	C: We [the caregiver and her husband] can get out for an hour, two hours; we would love to get out for, like, a couple of days, like overnight even, but we don't really have anybody out there. [People suggest] "phone your health care nurse, or phone home care; they'll come in and do the needles," but when you phone home care, they don't have the, the funds available to send anybody out.	

Table 3.1

CATEGORIES OF NONSUPPORTIVE INTERACTIONS WITH EXAMPLES *(continued)*

Caregiver Group and Situation		A = Woman Caring for Relative with Dementia B = Woman Caring for Relative/Friend with Cancer	C = Mother of Child with Diabetes or Asthma D = Mother of Infant Born Prematurely
Category	**Subcategory**	**Example Quotation by Caregiving Situation**	
		D: I really thought that there was more outside community help. . . . There is none, for all of the babies that I saw in there, row after row of these premature babies, there is not any premature baby groups, for the women to talk. I would have thought that there would have been something, somewhere.	
	Lack of connection to friends and family	B: You know, because it's [caregiving] a very isolating thing. My mom talked to me, and at times that meant that I walked away having had a conversation with my mother, that I didn't know what to do with.	
		C: So you tend to sort of distance yourself. At least, that's what we had to do. You distance yourself from a lot of family gatherings and stuff like this, which is kind of hard.	
	3.5 Promised help is not realized	A: They [relatives] offered to help, at the beginning, when Mom went in the nursing home, and when they took over to, to do the laundry, instead of getting it back the next day, 'cause she only had limited amount of clothes, they didn't get that for a week. So you can't rely on them, to do things to help. So you might as well do it yourself.	
		C: It's more aggravating, more stressful for me, if they offer to help, then don't follow through. 'Cause, it's very stressful, because you're relying on it. And when you go and get your heart set on something, it's like, oh, I'm gonna get where I don't have to worry about anything, and then it comes all crashing down around your head.	

believed that the other person was not listening, did not care, or was just interested in gossip. Some felt that if the query were genuine and potential helpers were really concerned, they would offer assistance.

> They'll phone and say "What's happening? Are you on top of this? What did Mom say? Have you noticed that Mom . . . ?" But they would never say "Would it be OK if I took Mom to the doctor?" (**Caregiver for her mother, who has dementia**)

Perspectives on what was nonsupportive could change over time, however. One mother, whose son had diabetes, noted that inquiries without offers of help were a problem when her son was first diagnosed but, later on, were positive for her.

Most forms of nonsupportive interactions were present in the four caregiving situations and in relationships with family and friends (informal social network), as well as with health and social service professionals (formal social network). We determined the presence or absence of each form of support and its subcategories in each caregiving situation and type of social network. The results of this are displayed in Table 3.2.

Caregivers in all situations described intimidation (Table 3.2, line 1.4) in their interactions with health and social service professionals, but not with family and friends. In contrast, they described a lack of support from family or friends who felt intimidated by caregiving demands (line 3.2) but did not perceive professionals as intimidated by the demands. There were a few variations between caregiving situations: Caregivers of a relative with dementia did not report blame (1.2) or unrealized promises of help from professionals (3.5), women caring for someone with cancer did not report unrealized promises of help from professionals (3.5), and mothers of infants born prematurely did not report having conflict with professionals (3.3).

Conditions Influencing Appraisal of Interactions

In monitoring and reflecting on interactions as supportive or nonsupportive, caregivers considered personal expectations and situational characteristics of their circumstances, as well as the nature of their social networks. In our study of women in four diverse caregiving situations, women were cognizant in their reflections of the influence of their personal expectations and feelings, as well as the attitudes of organizations

Table 3.2

PRESENCE OF NONSUPPORTIVE INTERACTIONS IN THE FORMAL AND INFORMAL SOCIAL NETWORKS OF CAREGIVERS

CATEGORY AND SUBCATEGORY OF NONSUPPORTIVE INTERACTIONS	GROUP A Relative with Dementia		GROUP B Relative/ Friend with Cancer		GROUP C Child with Diabetes or Asthma		GROUP D Infant Born Prematurely	
Social Network	F	I	F	I	F	I	F	I
1.0 Negative								
1.1 Discounting	Y	Y	Y	Y	Y	Y	Y	Y
1.2 Blaming	N	Y	Y	Y	Y	Y	Y	Y
1.3 Refusing to give support	Y	Y	Y	Y	Y	Y	Y	Y
1.4 Intimidating	Y	N	Y	N	Y	N	Y	N
1.5 Disrespecting	Y	Y	Y	Y	Y	Y	Y	Y
2.0 Ineffective								
2.1 Inadequate information	Y	Y	Y	Y	Y	Y	Y	Y
2.2 Inappropriate advice	Y	Y	Y	Y	Y	Y	Y	Y
2.3 Other inadequate/ inappropriate gestures of support	Y	Y	Y	Y	Y	Y	Y	Y
3.0 Absence of Expected Support								
3.1 Need is unrecognized	Y	Y	Y	Y	Y	Y	Y	Y
3.2 Helper is intimidated	N	Y	N	Y	N	Y	N	Y
3.3 No potential for support as a result of conflict	Y	Y	Y	Y	Y	Y	Y	Y
3.4 Help is not available	Y	Y	Y	Y	Y	Y	Y	Y
3.5 Promised help is not realized	N	Y	N	Y	Y	Y	Y	Y

Y = yes   F = Formal Social Network
N = no   I = Informal Social Network

or communities with which they interacted. As one woman noted, "It just depends."

In a second phase of the research, we presented women who had participated in earlier interviews, as well as some women who were being interviewed for the first time, with statements from earlier interviews with women—for their comments and classification of the statements as helpful or unhelpful. Women talked aloud about their rationale for the way they classified the statements in the context of their personal experience. These interviews were tape recorded.

Their comments reflected changing perspectives and divergence in interpretation that may occur with differences in context. Women repeatedly conveyed the personal expectation that they should maintain control of the care of their relative. They described this expectation in response to the invitation to comment on a statement made by other caregivers in an earlier interview, "They speak to others on my behalf."

> You still want to be in control . . . you still want to be the one who's being the caregiver. (**Caregiver for her mother, who has dementia**)

They felt that speaking on behalf of the caregiver should be done with the caregiver's permission and by someone they trusted.

> There [are] times that I don't feel comfortable with something, then having someone I trust . . . do it for me would be really nice. (**Caregiver for her mother, who has cancer**)

On the other hand, women acknowledged that they were willing for others to speak on their behalf when they were personally incapacitated by stress, ill health, or overwhelming demands.

> Oh, yeah, when I had my breakdown. I couldn't handle any more on my plate at that time. (**Mother of a child with diabetes**)

Some caregivers perceived pervasive attitudes in organizations or communities with which they interacted. These attitudes influenced their perceptions of what was supportive and nonsupportive. Two examples of the perspectives of others that women found to be nonsupportive were statements derived from initial interviews and presented to women for their comment in a later interview.

> Because the staff thought I was overprotective, they did not want to do as I asked.

Women in each of the four caregiving groups noted that staff in agencies caring for their relative thought they were overprotective and ignored their requests, resulting in potential for harm to their relative. A woman described how staff in the nursing home brushed off her request that her mother with dementia be assessed for a urinary infection. After she became upset, the test was done and her mother received treatment. The caregiver believed that she "was just this big irritation to them." Another participant, whose son had asthma, said:

> There are all these people who think, oh, you're just an overprotective mother. . . . You get it both from the professionals and in the community.

A woman caring for her husband who had cancer noted that she tried not to be overprotective, but staff thought they knew better than "the person that's been together [with the patient] for 40-some years."

Being considered overprotective had a positive outcome, however, for a daughter whose mother with dementia resided in a nursing home. She said:

> Staff have done the things I asked.

Caregivers explained that being perceived by staff as overprotective would be helpful when the staff knew more than they did, when their own emotions were interfering with the care needed by their relative, or when their actions were limiting the independence of their relative.

Some caregivers felt that their relative's appearance made it difficult to convince others that they needed help. When presented for their comments, the statement "My relative looks okay. Others don't know how ill he/she is" elicited comments that the appearance of well-being reinforced a perception that no special assistance or consideration was required.

> I would have given anything if anybody had realized how bad she was. (**Woman caring for a relative with dementia**)

A woman chastised one mother in a public mall for poking her diabetic daughter's finger to check her glucose level and then giving her an insulin injection.

> Because of [the caregiver's daughter's well-controlled] diabetes, a lot of people don't realize that she's sick.

At times, however, the appearance of well-being helped the child or adult feel normal and avoid pity from others. Mothers of children in school particularly felt that it was helpful that other children did not realize their child was ill and accepted their child as normal. One mother arranged for a special meal for their asthmatic son at a family wedding and placed him between his brothers to avoid awkwardness.

Consequences of Nonsupportive Interactions

In response to nonsupportive interactions, caregivers experienced negative feelings, such as anger, a loss of confidence in helpers, a loss of control, and a sense of powerlessness. Some caregivers modified their expectations, but others lost valued relationships. Many caregivers, however, reacted to nonsupportive interactions by becoming advocates for their relatives, in order to secure additional support and resources. The response of becoming an advocate is described more fully in Chapter 7.

Women

Women caring for a relative with dementia expressed anger in response to nonsupportive interactions. A few women caregivers expressed anger in response to nonsupportive interactions with either family and friends or professionals. For example, a daughter experienced anger when dealing with the staff of a long-term care facility.

> A lot of anger . . . I had asked them [the long-term care staff] to call the doctor, and they said he didn't come. In reality, they had not called him.

A granddaughter was very upset with the way her grandmother was treating her grandfather:

> She [her grandmother] could afford to give him any lifestyle he wanted, [but she did not] . . . and that made me really angry.

Angry feelings also arose for a mother who felt that her feelings had been disregarded when her premature twins were transferred to another hospital without consultation with her.

> *Nurse:* Your babies are moving. The ambulance is gonna be here in half an hour . . .
> *Mother:* What condition are they really in?

The mother went on to say that she felt like crying all the way over to the other hospital and that she thought the parents should have at least 8 hours notice.

A woman whose son had asthma described a loss of confidence in the treatment measures available to her son. She began to think that some intervention situations were hazardous rather than helpful to her son.

> We realize that . . . sometimes the interventions were not helpful for him. We didn't know why necessarily or understand . . . I almost started making a short list of places I wouldn't go and people I wouldn't see and situations he couldn't be in.

Another mother, whose child had asthma and severe allergies, lost confidence in teachers in her child's school. She was concerned they would ignore risks to her child.

> Some of the teachers, I am sure, thought, "She's nuts, and we aren't going to worry about [the child's allergies]."

A sense of losing control and a sense of powerlessness were particularly difficult for caregivers when confronting situations that were potentially life threatening for their relative, such as terminal cancer or allergies. One woman described her struggle to get staff to provide pain medication for her mother, who was dying of cancer and in pain.

> It was horrible, you know, feeling like . . . it was a great effort to get them to give her morphine . . . And I'm a firm believer . . . when you are dying you should die without pain as much as possible.

The mother of a child with asthma, who previously described her loss of confidence in staff, also noted her sense of powerlessness and despair.

You feel totally abandoned and isolated . . . You just go home and say . . . What am I supposed to do with this child? . . . We don't have any more resources here and we have no more answers. Where do we go? . . . You don't want to get too despairing about it, but there are times when you are.

Not all caregivers responded with anger, a loss of confidence, or a sense of powerlessness and loss of control. Sometimes caregivers modified expectations that were unfulfilled. A woman reduced her expectations for support from her son because she anticipated that her daughter-in-law would object, creating marital problems for her son. In other examples, caregivers decreased their expectations of adult children who had heavy responsibilities for parenting or work, were geographically distant, or had limited time or financial resources. This woman modified her expectations for support from her two sons.

Ron, he has left the city. Jim is very busy with his job, and he's got evening classes; he wants to work himself up, and I give him credit for that. So they don't really have time for me.

For some caregivers, the response to nonsupportive interactions was a loss of valued relationships. A woman who had formerly been the hub of family celebrations and interaction lost that family contact when the family withdrew as a result of disagreements over her decision to care for her grandfather in her home.

I've always been this—the nucleus of the family, the social convener . . . who always pulls everybody together and because they [her relatives] have had difficulty with even facing us, that's all falling apart.

Another woman in the same study described a loss of friendship relationships when the support that she expected was absent. Because her friends were unable to relate to the behavior changes occurring in her husband, who had dementia, she no longer participated in social activities and lost contact with them.

They [friends] don't seem to know what to say. And when they do come, and John seems disinterested or he's talking in a way that they can't understand, they just hesitate to come back. You're just completely overlooked when it comes to something that is couple-oriented.

Less frequently, women terminated relationships in response to nonsupportive interactions:

> I had girlfriends who didn't even call to ask me how she [her daughter] was . . . I no longer associate with those people.

Men

Although women were the primary focus of our research on nonsupportive interactions, examples of descriptions of nonsupportive interactions by men in our study of men caring for a relative with dementia suggest that their experiences may be similar to those of women and warrant further study. For example, a man caring for his wife with dementia described the nonsupportive behaviors of their children.

> I have more support in the Centre [a long-term care facility] than I do from my own family . . . that's the part that bloody well hurts. The boy hasn't been up in a year and a half to see his mother. My daughter hasn't been up since Christmas. [It was June at the time of the interview.] I'll be damned if I'll get on the phone.

Similarly, some men who had little interaction with or assistance from members of their family, whether they were distant or close, accepted the status quo and relinquished their expectations of aid by acknowledging that family members had other commitments.

DISCUSSION

Forms of Nonsupportive Interactions in Other Research

Reports of nonsupportive interactions in other research studies provide further support for the types of nonsupportive interaction that we identified—negative, ineffective, and absent. Moreover, such reports confirm the presence of similar forms of nonsupportive interactions in varied caregiving situations.

Negative Forms of Nonsupportive Interactions

Examples of negative nonsupportive interactions—in the form of minimizing, blaming, refusal to provide requested support, and disrespect—were reported in the literature on caregiving. Minimizing by professionals, family, and friends was identified in studies of parents whose child had a chronic condition (Gibson, 1995; Swallow & Jacoby 2001) and of adults caring for a relative dying at home from cancer (Stajduhar, 2003). In one study professionals implied blame when they suggested that mothers of a child with diabetes were "messing up" (Sullivan-Bolyai et al., 2003). Caregivers and their relatives with cancer experienced refusal of requests when they sought support from physicians for a peaceful death, but the physicians refused to provide this assistance (Meeker, 2004). Parents were refused requested support when day care staff would not accept children with type 1 diabetes despite state and federal laws making them eligible (Sullivan-Bolyai et al., 2003). Disrespect from health care providers was also found in studies of parents of a child with various chronic conditions (Kirschbaum & Knafl, 1996; Looman, 2004; Stewart, Hart, & Mann, 1995) and research on caregivers of adults with cancer (Meeker, 2004). In these studies, parents resented disrespectful interactions when they believed that they had experiential expertise, and caregivers of individuals with cancer reported that professionals failed to respect human dignity.

Ineffective Interactions

Interactions involving ineffective support have been reported among caregivers of adults with cancer in the form of inadequate information or support from professionals. Examples include caregivers of a relative with cancer not receiving information from health professionals about their relative's condition or the choices available (Meeker, 2004) or experiencing inadequate support from home care staff when their relative was dying of cancer (Stajduhar, 2003).

Absence of Expected Support. Research with similar caregiving populations has also reported examples of interactions comparable to our findings of the absence of support in relationships in which it was expected but absent. The failure of professionals to recognize caregivers' needs, for example, was reported in a study of mothers of children with type 1 diabetes, in which hospital staff did not recognize the mother's need for more information on care and problem solving (Sullivan-Bolyai et al., 2003). As in our research, according to which relatives or friends were sometimes intimidated by the caregiving demands, Sullivan-Bolyai et al. (2002, 2003) reported that grandmothers of a child with type 1 diabetes were afraid of their inability to respond if their diabetic grandchild developed hypoglycemia, and family and friends who initially offered to help were later unavailable or unwilling to fulfill their promise and provide assistance. Another example of the absence of expected support was reported by Meeker (2004) in a study of caregivers of dying relatives. Conflict among family members over the caregiver's choices for their relative dying of cancer resulted in absence of expected support for the caregiver.

Family research on dyadic coping in partners has similarly identified forms of nonsupportive interactions that were ambivalent, hostile, or superficial (Rafaeli & Gleason, 2009). Rafaeli and Gleason also suggest that actions intended to be helpful but fail to give assistance should be added to nonsupportive interactions. This latter type of nonsupport is similar to the category of ineffective actions identified in our research.

Theoretical Perspective

Women in our research described being family caregivers as an experience in which their understanding of supportive and nonsupportive interactions was influenced by their expectations and the resources in their social network. As the comment "It all depends" indicated, a key component of women's appraisal of interactions as supportive or nonsupportive was the fit between their specific requirements and expectations, in terms of resources and acceptable conditions for receiving aid, and the assistance offered or available within their environment.

Variations in the responses of women caregivers illustrate how personal beliefs and characteristics of a woman's social environment shaped her interactions with family, friends, and professionals and her reflection on whether these interactions were supportive. The quality of personal relationships with family and friends affected whether women were willing for others to act on their behalf. Relationships based on trust were perceived as supportive; relationships with conflict or feelings of distrust were viewed as nonsupportive. Social exchange theory predicts that women would seek assistance from those with whom they have a history of reciprocal exchange (Cook & Rice, 2003; Molm, Peterson, & Takahashi, 1999; Molm, Quist, & Wisely, 1994) because the exchange of support over time between family members or friends builds trust between the individuals. If support does not materialize when it is expected in a relationship, or the costs of receiving the support are perceived as too high, social exchange theory predicts that the relationship between the individuals will deteriorate.

The findings of our studies on nonsupport fit these predictions from social exchange theory. Women sought assistance from those in their informal social network who had exchanged support in the past, particularly those who signaled a willingness to help. When women's expectations of aid from these individuals were unfulfilled, they experienced their interactions with these individuals as nonsupportive. This occurred when offers of support and the assistance provided were inappropriate, as well as when support was absent, withdrawn, or provided with negative or demeaning comments.

The experiences of women caregivers with professionals and health care staff also support the theoretical premises of exchange theory. We argued in earlier chapters (e.g., Chapter 1) that the relationships between family caregivers and professionals or community agencies can be described as an example of negotiated exchanges. Negotiated exchanges involve the division of a finite pool of resources, and some individuals have more control over valued resources, such as nursing staff in comparison to family caregivers (Cook & Rice, 2003; Molm, Peterson, & Takahashi, 1999; Molm, Quist, & Wisely, 1994). In this type of relationship, there are greater costs to the individual with less power or fewer resources. Family caregivers who described difficulties in negotiating their role with nursing staff in caring for a family member in long-term care saw themselves as losing control and viewed the staff as nonsupportive. Professionals were viewed as nonsupportive when they did not provide the type of assistance that family caregivers expected, or when they made negative or disparaging comments about a caregiver's knowledge or contribution to the care of their relative. In these relationships, caregivers had relinquished control over the care of their family member in return for expectations of support but encountered greater costs than expected.

An ecological perspective also can facilitate understanding of the responses of women caregivers because it directs our attention to the interdependence of people and their environments and recognizes that environmental context may include multiple influential systems, such as the broader social or cultural environments (Trickett & Buchanan, 2001). Perceptions of social expectations were evident in the findings. Daughters expected that they would control care for their mothers, and their expectation is consistent with social expectations of what it means to be a good daughter (McCarty, 1996). Institutions such as hospitals, nursing homes, and schools have protocols for patients and students that can challenge a caregiver's goals and expectations for support. In care facilities, for example, the pervasive attitude of staff—that family caregivers are overprotective—conflicted with women's expectations to be in control of their relative's care and affected caregivers' perceptions of interactions as supportive or nonsupportive. Age-specific behavioral expectations of teachers, students, and other parents may indirectly contribute to stigma associated with disease or disability in a school-age child. For women, the experience of family caregiving included restructuring their social networks and redefining their expectations for support within a new and complex environment that included multiple levels of influence.

Our findings on nonsupportive interactions demonstrate that women were reflective about their own behavior and the actions of others, framing diverse viewpoints depending on their circumstances. Through a cyclical reflective process, they sought to regain control and to mobilize effective care for their relative and support for themselves. This cycle of reflecting and acting is congruent with an empowerment process described by Carr (2003), who reported that women made changes in themselves and their environment when faced with a challenging situation that contributed to a sense of powerlessness. In our research, nonsupportive interactions while caregiving was the stimulus for change.

Although our research on nonsupportive interactions was primarily with women, men caregivers' descriptions of nonsupportive interactions while caring for a relative with dementia suggest that their experience may be similar (Neufeld & Harrison, 1998). Men are continuing to assume family caregiving roles more frequently and may increasingly describe experiences similar to those of women. Findings from our study of men caregivers of a relative with dementia (not included in this book) further confirmed men's experience of nonsupportive interactions (Neufeld & Kushner, 2009). Research with other populations of men caregivers (Davies et al., 2004; McNeill, 2004) also suggests that these types of nonsupportive interactions are present among men caregivers.

We have considered women's experience of powerlessness and subsequent effort to make changes that restore their control in the context of social expectations for the role of women as good daughters or mothers and caregivers. An alternative explanation, congruent with identification of similar experiences among men, is the view that the lack of power and search for control that caregivers engage in is related primarily to the nature of negotiated exchanges, in which caregivers are powerless to secure the resources required for their relatives.

In conclusion, we have identified three forms of nonsupportive interactions that were present in the experience of women in different family caregiving situations. Women's perceptions of nonsupportive interactions were rooted in their expectations of support from family, friends, and professionals and in the social environment of their caregiving situation. We also documented the presence of similar nonsupportive interactions in the experience of men caring for a relative, usually their spouse, with dementia. We suggest that a social exchange perspective, focusing on the exchange of support in reciprocal relationships and the nature of negotiated exchange relationships, can be used by professionals to facilitate their understanding of caregivers' experience of nonsupportive interactions.

NOTE

The data reported in this chapter were drawn from the studies of women and men caregivers that were reported in the following publications: Fudge, Neufeld, & Harrison (1997); Harrison, Neufeld, & Kushner (1995); Neufeld, & Harrison (1998); Neufeld, & Harrison (2003); and Neufeld, Harrison, Hughes, & Stewart (2007). Primary emphasis is given to studies of nonsupportive interactions with women caregivers, particularly in Neufeld & Harrison (2003) and Neufeld et al. (2007).

REFERENCES

Carpentier, N., & Ducharme, F. (2005). Support network transformations in the first stages of the caregiver's career. *Qualitative Health Research, 15*(3), 289–311.

Carr, E. S. (2003). Rethinking empowerment theory using a feminist lens: The importance of process. *Affilia, 18*(1), 8–20.

Cohen, S. (2004). Social relationships and health. *American Psychologist, 59*(8), 676–684.

Cook, K. S., & Rice, E. (2003). Social exchange theory. In J. Delamater (Ed.), *Handbook of social psychology* (pp. 53–76). New York: Kluwer Academic/Plenum.

Davies, B., Gudmunsdottir, M., Worden, B., Orloff, S., Sumner, L., & Brenner, P. (2004). "Living in the dragon's shadow": Fathers' experiences of a child's life-limiting illness. *Death Studies, 28*, 111–135.

Fudge, H., Neufeld, A., & Harrison, M. J. (1997). Social networks of women caregivers. *Public Health Nursing, 14*(1), 20–27.

Gibson, C. H. (1995). The process of empowerment in mothers of chronically ill children. *Journal of Advanced Nursing, 21*, 1201–1210.

Harrison, M. J., Neufeld, A., & Kushner, K. (1995). Women in transition: Access and barriers to social support. *Journal of Advanced Nursing, 21*, 858–864.

Kirschbaum, M. S., & Knafl, K. A. (1996). Major themes in parent provider relationships: A comparison of life threatening and chronic illness experiences. *Journal of Family Nursing, 2*, 195–216.

Looman, W. S. (2004). Defining social capital for nursing: Experiences of family caregivers of children with chronic conditions. *Journal of Family Nursing, 10*, 412–428.

McCarty, E. (1996). Caring for a parent with Alzheimer's disease: Process of daughter caregiver stress. *Journal of Advanced Nursing, 23*, 792–803.

McNeill, T. (2004). Fathers' experience of parenting a child with juvenile rheumatoid arthritis. *Qualitative Health Research, 21*, 526–545.

Meeker, M. A. (2004). Family surrogate decision making at the end of life: Seeing them through with care and respect. *Qualitative Health Research, 14*, 204–225.

Molm, L. D., Peterson, G., & Takahashi, N. (1999). Power in negotiated and reciprocal exchange. *American Sociological Review, 64*, 876–890.

Molm, L., Quist, T. M., & Wisely, P. A. (1994). Imbalanced structures, unfair strategies: Power and justice in social exchange. *American Sociological Review, 59*, 98–121.

Neufeld, A., & Harrison, M. J. (1998). Men as caregivers: Reciprocal relationships or obligation? *Journal of Advanced Nursing, 28*(5), 959–968.

Neufeld, A., & Harrison, M. J. (2003). Unfulfilled expectations and negative interaction: Nonsupport in the relationships of women caregivers. *Journal of Advanced Nursing, 41*(4), 323–331.

Neufeld, A., Harrison, M. J., Hughes, K., & Stewart, M. (2007). Nonsupportive interactions in the experience of women family caregivers. *Health and Social Care in the Community, 15*(6), 530–541.

Neufeld, A., & Kushner, K. (2009). Men family caregivers' experience of nonsupportive interactions: Context and expectations. *Journal of Family Nursing, 15*(2), 171–191.

Pesiah, C., Brodaty, H., & Quadrio, C. (2006). Family conflict in dementia: Prodigal sons and black sheep. *International Journal of Geriatric Psychiatry, 21*, 485–492.

Rafaeli, E., & Gleason, M. E. J. (2009). Skilled support within intimate relationships. *Journal of Family Theory & Review, 1*, 20–37.

Ray, L. (2002). Parenting and childhood chronicity: Making visible the invisible work. *Journal of Pediatric Nursing, 17*(6), 424–438.

Stajduhar, K. I. (2003). Examining the perspectives of family members involved in the delivery of palliative care at home. *Journal of Palliative Care, 19*(1), 27–35.

Stewart, M. J., Hart, J., & Mann, K. V. (1995). Living with hemophilia and HIV/AIDS: Support and coping. *Journal of Advanced Nursing, 22*(6), 1101–1111.

Sullivan-Bolyai, S., Deatrick, J., Gruppuso, P., Tamborlane, W., & Grey, M. (2002). Mothers' experiences raising young children with type 1 diabetes. *Journal for Specialists in Pediatric Nursing, 7*, 93–103.

Sullivan-Bolyai, S., Deatrick, J., Gruppuso, P., Tamborlane, W., & Grey, M. (2003). Constant vigilance: Mothers' work parenting young children with type 1 diabetes. *Journal of Pediatric Nursing, 18*, 21–29.

Swallow, V. M., & Jacoby, A. (2001). Mothers' evolving relationships with doctors and nurses during the chronic illness trajectory. *Journal of Advanced Nursing, 36*, 755–764.

Trickett, E. J., & Buchanan, R. M. (2001). The role of personal relationships in transitions: Contributions of an ecological perspective. In B. Sarason & S. Duck (Eds.), *Personal relationships: Implications for clinical and community psychology* (pp. 141–157). New York: Wiley.

Wuest, J., Ericson, P. K., Stern, P. N., & Irwin G. W., Jr. (2001). Connected and disconnected support: The impact on caregiving support in Alzheimer's disease. *Health Care for Women International, 22*, 115–130.

Mobilizing Support from Family and Friends

Although social support may be available to caregivers from family and friends or professional sources within their social network, limited attention has been given to how caregivers mobilize support. Our research explored the preferences that guided caregivers' choices, the strategies they used, and the barriers that they addressed when seeking to establish a helpful source of aid. In this chapter we address how caregivers monitored their relationships with family and friends and sought to mobilize support from these sources within their networks. The support that participants sought included emotional, physical, and informational support (Dunkel-Schetter, Folkman, & Lazarus, 1987). We address mobilization of support from professionals and organizations in Chapter 5.

SOCIAL EXCHANGE THEORY

We conducted our research on support mobilization using the perspective of social exchange theory (Cook & Rice, 2003) to examine family caregivers' preferences for the sources of their support and their deliberation when seeking support. As a foundation for mobilizing support, family caregivers carefully monitor their caregiving situation. This process includes monitoring and reflecting on the health status of their relative and their relative's need for care, as well as reflecting on the relationships that caregivers and their relative have with friends, family members, and health professionals. Consistent with social exchange theory, caregivers in our research monitored reciprocity, the exchange of support in relationships with friends and family. In relationships with professionals, they monitored mutuality or collaboration and patterns of interaction over time.

We included both collective and individual orientations in exchange theory (Sabatelli & Shehan, 1993). A collective exchange perspective encompasses the understanding that different social norms and expectations of reciprocity exist for different types of relationships. For example, caregivers might expect more support or different types of support from family members than from friends. These expectations would be based on the norms and values held by their family and their community. The individualistic exchange perspective assumes that individuals calculate personal costs and rewards and consider alternatives before acting. Costs and risks in seeking help may include loss of self-esteem, loss of privacy, the perception of indebtedness, and uncertainty about the response of the other (Goldsmith & Parks, 1990; Molm, Takahashi, & Peterson, 2000), and individuals weigh these costs against the value of the support that they might receive. In addition, the support an individual receives can be accompanied by strain and conflict in relationships (Rook, 1990; Wuest, Ericson, Stern, & Irwin, 2001). As we discussed in Chapter 3, on nonsupport, caregivers might accept offers from a family member to assist in caring for a senior with dementia but know that the helper will continue to argue with them over the need for respite services or that the helper may criticize how the caregiver has arranged for homemaker assistance. Social exchange theory predicts that caregivers who view support as helpful and available at little cost or risk will be more likely to use it than those who perceive a high cost in relation to the support that is received.

Monitoring and Reflecting

Implicit in the perspective of social exchange theory is the act of monitoring relationships over time, as part of the process of considering alternatives in giving and seeking support. In the context of family caregiving, caregivers reflect on the health condition of their relative, the care that is needed, and the support that the caregiver may require to provide the care. Research indicates that caregivers are vigilant in their efforts to watch over their premature infants (Hurst, 2001), to monitor symptoms of a child with special needs (Ray, 2002), or to observe changes in their relative with dementia (Bowers, 1987, 1988; Heinrich, Neufeld, & Harrison, 2003). As caregivers monitor, interpret, and reflect on their situation, they consider the potential for support in their relationships with kin and friends and their connections with professional sources of assistance, as well as the health condition and care needed by the care recipient. In our research, we incorporated an examination of how caregivers monitored the relationships that were potentially supportive.

Relationship between Informal and Formal Sources of Support

Because family caregivers rely on informal support from friends and family, as well as from formal or professional sources, we assumed an integrative perspective that incorporates both sources within a caregiver's social network (Carpentier & Ducharme, 2003). Although there is general consensus that caregivers rely on assistance from both sources, divergent theoretical perspectives exist on the ways in which professional and kin/friend sources of support intersect within family caregiving situations (Dupuis & Norris, 1997; Penning, 2002). As a foundation for discussion of mobilizing support, we next discuss theoretical perspectives on the relationship between informal and formal sources of support.

Some theorists have suggested that professional services may substitute for the efforts of family caregivers when the latter are unavailable or insufficient. Sometimes referred to as the hierarchical-compensatory model (Cantor, 1975; Lyons & Zarit, 1999), this traditional view suggests that close relatives are the preferred source of support for an individual with a health problem and that professional assistance is sought only when family support is unavailable. The task-specific model, however, suggests that different forms of assistance are sought from informal and professional sources (Litwak, 1985; Lyons & Zarit, 1999; Penning, 2002). From this latter perspective, family members are best able to provide for everyday needs and emotional support, whereas professional sources are better able to provide specialized or technical forms of assistance. These two views are overlapping, but both are limited in their acknowledgment of the dynamic nature of social networks and the fluctuating, multiple sources of assistance.

If support for an individual with a health issue can be obtained informally from family and friends, or formally from professionals and paraprofessionals, what guides the family caregiver's selection of a source of support for themselves? Are the models outlined previously appropriate to examine support for family caregivers? If a family caregiver's choice of source of support is based on the closeness of the relationship, as proposed by the hierarchical-compensatory model (Cantor, 1975), the preferred order for the selection of the helper begins with the spouse, followed by other relatives, then friends and neighbors, and finally formal sources such as professionals or organizations. The latter sources of help are used as substitutes in the absence of preferred sources of help—that is, family and close friends.

A focus on the nature of the connection between family and professional sources of assistance in family caregiving has sometimes been accompanied by the belief that reliance on professional sources of aid may undermine self-reliance and family responsibility. The results of a study of the extent of professional assistance in home care, self-care, and family care among older adults with chronic illness and disability, including some with cognitive impairment, suggested, however, that professional services for these adults were not a substitute for family assistance. Instead, as levels of illness and disability increased, increased assistance from all sources was required (Penning, 2002).

The selection of a source of support can, however, be made by matching the nature of the support needed in caregiving with the characteristics of the potential helping group, as identified in the task-specific model (Allen & Ciambrone, 2003; Litwak, 1985). For example, the informal system of family and friends can assist with unpredictable, nonuniform, nontechnical caregiving tasks, whereas the formal system manages specialized, predictable tasks, and the two systems complement one another by virtue of their task specificity.

According to another perspective (Edelman & Hughes, 1990), the supplementary model, the formal system supplements the informal system, not according to particular tasks but when the needs of the care recipient exceed the resources of the informal system. This perspective is similar to that of the complementary model (Chappell & Blandford, 1991), in which formal care is used when elements of the informal system are insufficient, and formal care may compensate for this, or when the informal network is adequate, but the need is very high, and supplementary assistance is required. From this latter perspective, family caregivers would seek support from the health care system when they and their family and friends were unable to provide adequate care for their relative.

Social Network Ties

One of the conditions influencing how family caregivers mobilize support from kin and friends is the nature of the caregivers' social network ties. *Social network* has been defined as a web of social ties that surround an individual (Berkman, 1984). These ties can be continuous or intermittent over time. Research on social networks has often focused on such characteristics as size (number of members); strength of ties; density (links between members); homogeneity of membership in terms of characteristics such as gender, age, or relationship; and dispersion of members (Berkman, Glass, Brissette, & Seeman, 2000; Cohen, Teresi, & Blum, 1994; Walker, MacBride, & Vachon, 1977). In our research, we used ecomaps (Wright & Leahy, 2005) to provide a graphic portrayal of family caregivers' social relationships and the nature of their ties with others (Hartman, 1995), as well as changes in caregivers' social networks over time. Ecomaps are a method of diagrammatically indicating members of a social network, using circles to indicate members and lines and arrows to indicate the nature of connections. We discuss our use of ecomaps in research in more depth in Chapter 9. We also used the Arizona Social Support Interview Schedule (ASSIS), (Barrera, 1981; Barrera & Baca, 1990) to facilitate differentiation among ties that were conflicted and those that were either potential or utilized sources of support.

MOBILIZING SUPPORT FROM FAMILY AND FRIENDS

In our research on mothers facing a life transition (Harrison & Neufeld, 1997; Harrison, Neufeld, & Kushner, 1995) and on family caregivers (Neufeld & Harrison, 1995), we learned that individuals have specific preferences for their source of support and that they prefer to accept offers of support rather than ask for support. In the following sections of this chapter, we present our findings on support preferences, summarize the barriers to requesting support that were discussed by our research participants, and illustrate how characteristics of the social network influence the mobilization of social support.

Selecting an Acceptable Source of Support

There can be strong preferences for the source of support—based on emotional ties, kinship, or expertise—and the preferred source of support may change over time. These sources of support were described in a study of mothers experiencing a major life transition, such as birth of their first child or returning to work after an extended absence because of childrearing. The women preferred support that came from individuals who they viewed as sharing commitment, history, and close emotional ties in a relationship. Individuals who shared the experience of the life transition were the next preferred source of support. Women described their desire to obtain support by speaking with other individuals who were also new parents or survivors in the workplace after years of being at home childrearing. One mother commented about those who had not experienced the life transition.

> There just isn't that sort of common link there. They would think you were a bit odd [to ask for support].

Expertise in child care was important to the new mothers, and closer relationships developed with individuals who were seen as supportive in this area. The women who returned to work described the importance of relationships with coworkers and with other mothers who worked outside the home. Most informants preferred to get support from people; books provided a shared experience for only one woman.

> You can only get so much out of a book. And who has time to read it anyway? You know, you learn from other people's experiences.

Specialized sources of support, such as Alcoholics Anonymous or health professionals, were sought when the special expertise available from established community programs was required. Two women in the return-to-work group, who had very limited support from relationships with others who shared a close commitment or common experience, made the most use of specialized sources of support.

Offers of Support Reducing the Cost of Accepting Support

Caregivers preferred that support was offered to them rather than having to request it, and they were reluctant to seek assistance. Some individuals viewed requests for support as an admission of inadequacy or dependence.

> I always try to handle things on my own. I don't want to bother anybody; I feel like I'm whining again.

This woman's reluctance to ask for help reflected her belief that requests for help can be seen as unjustified complaints.

When support was offered to caregivers before they had to request it, barriers such as fear of refusal, diminished self-esteem, or concern about burdening the supporter were reduced. The caregivers described the use of volunteered support as a means of avoiding the costs associated with requesting support. A man caring for his wife with dementia described this sentiment:

> I can't ask for help. It's just not in my character. Where, if somebody offered, I would probably accept.

To avoid making requests for support, many employed strategies such as trying to do everything themselves, delaying requests until a crisis occurred, exhibiting nonverbal cues, or accepting offers of help when they were not needed to sustain the potential for assistance in the future. However, as one mother of a premature infant commented, waiting for support to be volunteered could result in difficulties in coping without support,

> I don't like to ask other people to do things for me. I will do them on my own if it kills me. So that leads to all kinds of problems.

A number of the new mothers and mothers returning to work delayed requesting help until the situation reached a crisis. Once they had decided that the situation was a crisis and more than they could be expected to manage, they considered it acceptable to ask for help.

One mother of a premature infant illustrated the use of behavioral cues. She was very concerned that if she asked for help, others would refuse, so she relied on nonverbal signals to communicate her need for support. Her use of nonverbal cues to signal the need for support was a strategy that enabled her to avoid asking for support. However, her reliance on nonverbal cues was limited to the period of the infant's hospitalization. Once her child was at home, she believed that her use of nonverbal cues to signal her distress had become inappropriate, but she was unable to ask for support directly in case her request was ignored or refused:

> I'm not giving them signs that I need help. Before, they could hear it in my voice, they could see it in my face when Amy was in hospital. Now Amy is 6 months old, and I don't let it show . . . because I don't want to get hurt.

A woman caring for her husband who had dementia described accepting offers whether she needed assistance at the time or not:

> I've learned if someone phones on a cold day and says, "Do you need some-thing at the store?" whether I need bread or not, I always say, "Oh, I'd sure like a loaf of brown bread." Whereas, perhaps two or three years ago, I would have said, "Oh, I'm fine. I don't need anything, thank you." But now if somebody does offer a specific thing I try really hard to say, "Yes I need it." Because then I think they might do it again.

This woman had learned to maintain relationships in which support was offered for times when she would need help. In this way, she reduced the costs of having to request support.

Barriers and Costs to Requesting Support for Women Caregivers

In research with women caring for a relative with dementia and with mothers of an infant born prematurely, we examined the barriers they considered in thinking about making a request for support from a friend or family member. The barriers that we identified are presented in Figure 4.1. We have presented the barriers in relation to the process of making a request for support. We chose a wheel to illustrate the pro-cess of requesting support because the caregivers described continuous evaluation of the barriers in relation to the phases of requesting support. The inner wheel represents the components in the process of requesting support (e.g., allow, acknowledge). The outer wheel represents the bar-riers associated with each component. In making decisions on whether to request support, an individual caregiver often focused on one or two barriers and seldom described a clear sequence in decision making. The barriers in Figure 4.1 are discussed in relation to each component of the process of requesting support. We begin with the components of allow and acknowledge and move clockwise around the wheel displayed in Figure 4.1.

Allow and Acknowledge

Before seeking support, it was necessary that caregivers be willing to allow others to assist them with caregiving and to acknowledge that assis-tance was needed. Some caregivers considered caregiving to be their

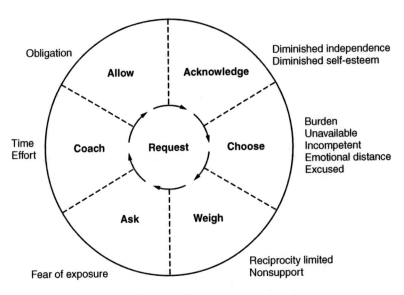

Figure 4.1. Barriers to requesting support.

personal obligation. They viewed themselves as responsible for the care recipient and were unwilling to share this responsibility with others. A woman caring for a relative with dementia noted:

> I wouldn't let someone else take over what I do because I need to.

A mother of an infant born prematurely commented:

> I'm the one that had the children, so I should be the one that takes care of them.

For some caregivers, having to ask for support meant acknowledging to themselves and others that they were incapable of providing care. They described diminished independence and self-esteem. Their caregiving role was a source of pride, and they were reluctant to admit, even to themselves, that they needed help.

> When you can't manage on your own, you feel like somehow you've failed, and so if you're a failure, you hate to point this out to someone else and ask for help. (**Mother of a premature infant**)

Choose

There were many barriers in the next phase of the process, choosing an acceptable source of support. Some caregivers did not ask for support because they thought their request would place a burden on others. They described carefully assessing the degree of burden their request would represent.

> It has to be something that I need to do really, really badly before I would ask anybody else to help, because I realize that everybody is busy with their own problems and nearly everybody has somebody sick or some reason that they can't do it. (**Woman caring for a relative with dementia**)

Some caregivers described in detail the degree of anticipated burden, and they took into account the length of time that they might require support, the amount of effort necessary to provide the specific type of support, other responsibilities of the potential helper, and the provider's resources of energy and health. For example, new mothers frequently made a careful assessment of their husband's work commitments and adjusted their expectations accordingly.

> I've already made up my mind, like I'm not going to pressure him to do things [with the baby or the house] if he has to do things related to his work.

Another woman decided, before the birth of her infant, that she could not ask for support from her mother because her father was ill and her parents were elderly; she was also reluctant to ask for help from colleagues at work unless she was totally strapped because they were busy working full-time.

For other caregivers, the support that they required was simply unavailable. Examples included family members who lived in another province, a potential helper who lacked financial resources, or an inability of the caregiver to access sources of information about community agencies. At times, family members and friends were viewed as incompetent and unable to provide support in caring for the infant or older adult.

Some sources of help were seen as unacceptable because of emotional distance; their relationship was not close enough in kinship or affinity. Caregivers expressed a strong preference for support to come from close family members or from friends who shared the same experience.

When this type of relationship existed, the caregivers felt that they could expect support. They were disappointed when others did not respond to their request for support. As one woman said,

> I was really disappointed with them [her friends] because I thought they were really close. (**Mother of a premature infant**)

In addition, caregivers sometimes excused potential supporters from providing assistance such as household help or substitute care. When someone was excused, caregivers implied that those individuals who were excused could help and might be expected to do so. However, they preferred to excuse them. For example, one woman explains why she would not ask her daughter to help:

> I wouldn't want to damage the relationship between her and her father, because when he was in the early stages [of decreased cognitive functioning] she was still at home, and it was difficult.

Mothers of premature infants frequently excused their husband from providing help with household duties.

> If he's lying on the couch with a very sleepy look on his face and says, "Don't worry, dear, I'll clean it up." I'll say, "No, don't worry about it," because I know his heart is not in it.

Weigh

Caregivers also weighed the costs of using support. As discussed in Chapter 2, they felt that reciprocity, or give-and-take, was important for the continuation of relationships. They were reluctant to seek support if they thought that they might be unable to reciprocate, because this could threaten the continuation of the relationship. One mother, in discussing child care, commented:

> I feel better when I can reciprocate the help than [when it is] a one-sided affair.

Women also considered the potential for nonsupportive interactions, as discussed in Chapter 3, as a cost of asking for aid. When nonsupport was anticipated, they often decided not to ask for help.

Ask

When caregivers were verbally asking for support, there was a fear of refusal, as well as a fear of exposure and loss of privacy. The caregivers were reluctant to provide detailed explanations for why they needed support.

> When you're asking for it [support], a lot of times you've got to tell them the reason why and go into great in-depth discussion about it. You can't just say, "Would you do this for me?" (**Mother of a premature infant**)

In providing detailed explanations, the caregivers experienced a loss of privacy that made them more vulnerable if their request for support was refused.

Coach

The time and effort needed to coach others to provide assistance and care may be too costly for caregivers. Women whose premature infants were on supplemental oxygen at home described the effort to train others to care for the infant when they wanted some relief from child care. For some mothers, the time and energy required for training exceeded the benefits of time free from child care. Women caring for an older adult sometimes refused assistance from homemakers because of the time and effort required to show the homemaker how to provide appropriate assistance.

Barriers and Costs to Requesting Support for Men Caregivers

Identification of the preceding barriers and costs to requesting support emerged in a study of the support experience of mothers of an infant born prematurely and women caring for a relative with dementia. We also analyzed data from a study of men caregivers and confirmed the presence of these barriers among men caring for a relative with dementia. For example, a man caring for his wife with dementia felt responsible for her care and did not want to allow others to assist him or acknowledge that assistance was needed.

> All the things I do on my own, I always figured was my responsibility, nobody else's.

Another man described his reluctance to admit the need for help and the negative personal feelings that would be associated with such a request.

> I would feel extremely badly about asking for help, but I would only do it as a last resort.

In choosing an acceptable source of support, assessing the degree of burden that their request could create for the helper is illustrated in the comment of a participant who was hesitant to ask his daughter for help:

> Well, I've got my daughter, but I hate to be phoning her all the time . . . because she is not well herself.

Men, like the women, were hesitant to request or accept support if they were unable to reciprocate. A man caring for his wife with dementia described his loss of social interaction with friends because he could not reciprocate and entertain.

> We used to have dinner together, you know. But, I can't invite anybody in and, ah 'cause I don't think it's fair to them . . . so I feel sort of hesitant about being entertained.

Men caring for a relative with dementia, similar to the women that we interviewed, feared exposure and loss of privacy when making a request for support. A man caring for his wife, who had dementia, explained it this way:

> At times I thought . . . why are they bothering me? Why are they infringing on my privacy?

The barriers described in the process of requesting support were similar for the caregivers caring for an infant born prematurely or a relative with dementia, although the examples varied, particularly in relation to the barrier of the time and the effort needed to coach others to provide assistance. For example, in relation to the time and effort needed to coach others to provide assistance, mothers referred to the effort necessary to prepare a babysitter to provide physical care for the premature infant, whereas women caring for older persons were often frustrated by the need to educate new homemakers repeatedly in the routines required. The effort required in coaching others to provide care was the only barrier to requesting support that was not evident in our interview data among men caregivers of a relative with dementia. All other barriers described were present for men or women caring for a relative with dementia, as well as for mothers of infants born prematurely.

Influence of the Nature of the Social Network in Mobilization of Support

We analyzed the relationship between social networks and the mobilization of support in a study of women caring for a relative with dementia. We gathered data using ecomaps, the Arizona Social Support Interview Schedule, and in-depth qualitative interviews to generate a typology representing patterns of women's social networks and the implications of these patterns for mobilization of support.

Typology of Social Networks

The patterns of membership of the social networks and characteristics of the individuals within the networks were portrayed in the form of a typology representing variations. The typology of social networks of the women caregivers is portrayed in Table 4.1. The typology was developed from extensive analysis of the interview data and confirmed by data in the ASSIS and ecomaps. Perceptions of conflict, satisfaction, and types of support received were then examined according to type of network.

Three distinct types of networks emerged: diverse networks, semi-diverse networks, and kin-focused networks. Diverse networks consisted of many different types of members. Incidences of conflict were rare, and satisfaction with the support received was high. Semi-diverse networks had fewer variations in the type and number of members. Incidences of conflict were more frequent, and not all caregivers were satisfied with the support provided. Kin-focused networks comprised primarily family members and a small number of friends. Conflict was frequent, and none of the caregivers reported satisfaction with the support that they received. The kinds of conflict caregivers experienced in their interactions with family and friends included a lack of concern for them or the care recipient, experiences of nonsupport, anger, dissatisfaction with support intended to assist the caregiver, and disagreements about how

Table 4.1

TYPOLOGY OF SOCIAL NETWORKS OF 20 WOMEN CAREGIVERS

Network Characteristics	SUPPORT NETWORK		
	Diverse ($n = 9$)	Semi-Diverse ($n = 7$)	Kin-Focused ($n = 4$)
Size	Large	Medium	Small
Range of members	Widely varied	Somewhat varied	Limited variation
Network members	Recipient	Recipient	Recipient
	Relatives	Relatives	Relatives
	Friends	Friends	Friends
	Professionals	Professionals	Professionals
	Support groups	Support groups	Support groups
	Social groups	Social groups	
	Church		
	Colleagues		
	Local business		
Proximity of network members	Some close	Some close	All close
	Some far	Some far	None far
Interconnectedness	Varied	Varied	Connected
Conflict	Occasional	Fairly frequent	Frequent
	Small amount	Moderate amount	Large amount
Satisfaction of caregiver	Most satisfied	Some satisfied	None satisfied

the caregivers or others treated the care recipient. Caregivers described some relationships in which there was only conflict and other relationships in which conflict and support coexisted.

Types of Support Present

Caregivers reported differences in the types and amount of support that they received. These differences varied in relation to the type of social network the caregiver had. The types of support described by the women caregivers and listed in Table 4.2 were instrumental, emotional (including appraisal), and informational.

As Table 4.2 indicates, there was variation in the frequency and category of support provided by the three types of networks. Those caregivers with diverse social networks received the most frequent and broadest range of social support, whereas those caregivers with kin-dominated social networks received support less often and experienced fewer kinds of support. Emotional support in the form of appraisal or feedback was

Table 4.2

CATEGORY AND FREQUENCY OF SUPPORT REPORTED BY NETWORK TYPE

	SUPPORT NETWORK		
Support Reported	Diverse (*n* = 9)	Semi-Diverse (*n* = 7)	Kin-Focused (*n* = 4)
Instrumental			
Labor	Frequently	Frequently	Rarely
Aid in kind	Sometimes	Rarely	Rarely
Money	Rarely	Never	Rarely
Modifying the environment	Rarely	Never	Never
Emotional			
Concern	Frequently	Sometimes	Rarely
Trust	Sometimes	Rarely	Rarely
Listening	Rarely	Rarely	Rarely
Affect	Rarely	Rarely	Rarely
Esteem	Rarely	Rarely	Rarely
Appraisal			
Social comparison	Rarely	Never	Rarely
Feedback	Rarely	Never	Never
Affirmation	Rarely	Rarely	Rarely
Information			
Information	Sometimes	Sometimes	Rarely
Advice	Rarely	Rarely	Rarely
Suggestions	Never	Rarely	Rarely

lacking from semi-diverse and kin-focused social networks. Emotional support, such as social comparison, feedback, and appraisal in the form of affirmation, demonstrated to the caregiver that other caregivers often experienced similar feelings and circumstances, and it also acknowledged the care given by the caregiver.

In conclusion, the type of social network of caregivers (diverse, semi-diverse, or kin-focused) was accompanied by differences in types of support experienced. Women with diverse networks were more content with the support they received than women with kin-dominated or semi-diverse networks. In addition, women's experience with conflict in relationships with network members and the degree and frequency with which the conflict occurred varied according to the type of social network.

DISCUSSION

With respect to the mobilization of support from family members and friends, a social exchange perspective encompasses the recognition that social norms and expectations for providing, accepting, and reciprocating support vary for different types of relationships. Because of their close family relationship to the care recipient, some women viewed their caregiving as an obligation. Their perception of this obligation required that they provide care without asking for support. Women also did not ask for support from someone unless they perceived the relationship with the potential sources of support to be sufficiently close.

The preference for receiving support—from those friends and family members with shared commitment and shared experience—and the emphasis placed on the ability to reciprocate support are consistent with social exchange theory (Cook & Rice, 2003). Social exchange theory postulates that any relationship that endures evolves into a reciprocal relationship and that individuals will leave relationships in which they consistently perceive inequitable returns (Molm, Quist, & Wisely, 1994). In intimate relationships, which caregivers described as their preferred sources of support, the exchange of support occurred over time, and there was no specific need for immediate reciprocity.

The inability to reciprocate support was a barrier to asking for help, whereas a history of give-and-take in exchange of support between individuals facilitated the ability to seek support. The women experiencing a normative life transition described relationships that included give-and-take, or the exchange of help in various forms. Their emphasis on the potential to provide future help to a supporter—or their assessment that the help that they gave previously enabled them to ask for help later—is evidence that they are part of reciprocal relationships.

One woman who perceived herself as unable to reciprocate the offers of help she received had the smallest social network and the most limited resources to share. She consistently described situations in which she refused assistance because she could not reciprocate. A small network is more common among older caregivers as they experience losses in relationships through illness or death (Carpentier & Ducharme, 2003). Others argue for a focus on care networks, which represent those directly involved in care of an individual with a health problem, as distinct from a dyad of a single caregiver and a care recipient, or broader social support networks that extend beyond individuals contributing to care of someone with a health problem (Keating, Otfinowski, Wenger, Fast, & Derksen, 2003). Our emphasis, however, includes the broader social network as a source of support for the caregiver.

Communal relationships, such as family ties and close friendships with others who share similar experiences, depend less on immediate reciprocity (Clark, Mills, & Powell, 1986). When many different types of problems and activities are shared, the relationship is stronger and provides more social support, particularly emotional support. Some researchers (Lin, Dumm, & Woelfel, 1986; Pyke & Bengston, 1996) have suggested that some families hold a strong view that there is a connection between close ties and eldercare, often refusing professional assistance. We discuss this perspective in more depth in Chapter 6, on family caregiving and mobilizing support during migration. Other families may hold more individualistic norms that value members' independence and facilitate acceptability of accepting professional assistance.

These examples show that norms or expectations for support vary in different types of relationships. These norms and expectations are related to larger social processes and structures. Although caregivers, like others, may continuously develop and revise expectations and perceptions in ongoing interactions with those around them (Murray, 2002), pervasive social norms continue to be influential. For example, the family norms that reward women for assuming primary responsibility in caregiving arise from larger social norms that label caregiving as women's work. Thompson (1991) has examined women's sense of fairness in family work. She argued that when women and their families accept that women do the lion's share of family work, such as caregiving, and that others "help women," necessary family work that should be the responsibility of all family members is turned into women's personal needs. In the context of this view, others' contributions are seen as a sacrifice beyond what could normally be expected—or as care for the woman—rather than an expected and appropriate contribution to the family work.

Our finding that some women excuse husbands and children from assisting with caregiving or household tasks to avoid putting a strain on a family relationships has also been identified by other researchers (Abel, 1989; Hochschild, 1989; Litt, 2004; Smith, Smith, & Toseland, 1991). There is no expectation that the work or responsibility of women will be shared with or given to others. By accepting responsibility within the family, these women decrease conflict within family relationships and do not challenge societal expectations for women's role in caregiving. However, this response limits the support available to women and may jeopardize their health as they struggle to provide care.

At the individual level, caregivers in our research described numerous costs of seeking support: a loss of privacy, decreased independence, decreased self-esteem, and perceived incompetence. Women avoided support that was accompanied by negative comments and conflict. They also used strategies to obtain support that avoided direct requests for aid. These findings support our argument that caregivers monitor relationships and weigh the costs and benefits of support before requesting assistance.

A cost associated with accepting support was the caregivers' perception that they were obligated to reciprocate. As a consequence of their adherence to a norm of reciprocity, caregivers were reluctant to ask for support unless they believed that they could return support within an acceptable time period. This view is analogous to a psychological "social support bank" (Antonucci & Jackson, 1990) from which withdrawals may be made because contributions have been given in the past or are anticipated in the future. An inability to reciprocate support may leave the caregiver with feelings of indebtedness and discomfort that inhibit requests for aid. Other researchers have also identified that individuals may feel indebted in accepting support (Bolger, Zuckerman, & Kessler, 2000), be reluctant to make direct requests for support and prefer that support be offered to them (Hayes, 2006). In addition, research with couples suggests that the receipt of support without reciprocation may undermine the recipient's sense of self-esteem or autonomy and imply that he or she is not capable (Bolger, Zuckerman, & Kessler, 2000; Rafaeli & Gleason, 2009).

Our analysis revealed that the process of ultimately requesting support involved consideration of a series of potential barriers to making a request for support that began with acknowledging the need for support and culminated in making the request for assistance. Although we did not label this process in terms of stages in seeking support, other research, guided by a stress and coping perspective, suggests three common stages in support transactions: initially identifying the stressor and associated needs, appraisal and communication of the need for support, and finally action (Rafaeli & Gleason, 2009). Even though our findings include a more detailed description of the issues or potential barriers that caregivers considered before requesting assistance, the experience of caregivers in our research is congruent with Rafaeli and Gleason's broader conceptualization of stages in support transactions.

Our findings of variation in the type of social networks that women caregivers of a relative with dementia exhibited and differences in their perceptions of support or conflict (Fudge, Neufeld, & Harrison, 1997) are also similar to those of other researchers (Lilly, Richards, & Buckwalter, 2003; Wenger, 1991). Wenger identified family-dependent, locally integrated, locally self-contained, wider community-focused, and private, restricted networks among elders in Wales. In our findings, diverse networks, similar to Wenger's locally integrated and wider community-focused networks, were better able to meet the needs of the caregivers. The presence of friends, which has been identified as a significant source of emotional and social integration support, is likely to be more evident in diverse networks of caregivers of a relative with dementia (Lilly et al., 2003). Wenger's family-dependent and private, restricted networks are similar in composition and ability to provide support to the kin-focused and semi-diverse networks in our research, respectively.

Less attention has been given to social networks and support seeking of men caregivers (Russell, 2007). Russell (2004) found that establishing social connections was difficult for men caregivers of spouses with dementia and that their opportunities to socialize were limited. In Wenger's (1991) typology of social networks among the elderly, single men were the most likely to have small networks, and men's networks shrank when their spouse died, whereas women's did not. We found, in a comparison of the social networks of men and women caring for a relative with dementia, that younger men and those of higher socioeconomic status reported larger available social networks than other men did and that, in comparison to men, women had larger conflicted social networks that comprised more family members (Hibbard, Neufeld, & Harrison, 1996). In an Australian study of barriers to support for community-dwelling co-resident caregivers of a relative with dementia, men and women caregivers experienced similar barriers to accessing support from services (Bruce & Paterson, 2000). In this study, the emphasis was on access to professional services rather than on support from family and friends

In conclusion, the findings presented in this chapter provide insight into the reflection and deliberation of caregivers as they seek to mobilize support from family and friends. Caregivers' preferences for access to support, their strategies in securing support, the barriers they consider, and the costs they incur in accepting assistance from others can inform professionals who seek to assist caregivers in securing assistance and guide family and friends as they interact with family caregivers.

NOTE

The data reported in this chapter were drawn from the studies of women and men caregivers that were reported in the following publications: Fudge, Neufeld, & Harrison (1997); Harrison & Neufeld (1997); Harrison, Neufeld, & Kushner (1995); Neufeld & Harrison (1994); and Neufeld & Harrison (1995).

REFERENCES

Abel, E. K. (1989). The ambiguities of social support: Adult daughters caring for frail elderly parents. *Journal of Aging Studies, 3,* 211–230.

Allen, S., & Ciambrone, D. (2003). Community care for people with disabilities: Blurring the boundaries between formal and informal caregivers. *Qualitative Health Research, 13,* 207–226.

Antonucci, T. C., & Jackson, J. S. (1990). The role of reciprocity in social support. In B. R. Sarason, I. G. Sarason, & G. R. Pierce (Eds.), *Social support: An interactional view* (pp. 173–198). New York: Wiley.

Barrera, M. (1981). Social support in the adjustment of pregnant adolescents: Assessment issues. *Social Networks and Social Support, 4,* 69–96.

Barrera, M., & Baca, L. M. (1990). Recipient reactions to social support: Contributions of enacted support and network orientation. *Journal of Social and Personal Relationships, 7*(4), 541–551.

Berkman, L. (1984). Assessing the physical health effects of social networks and social support. *Annual Review of Public Health, 5,* 413–432.

Berkman, L., Glass, T., Brissette, I., & Seeman, T. (2000). From social integration to health: Durkheim in the new millennium. *Social Science & Medicine, 51,* 843–857.

Bolger, N., Zuckerman, A., & Kessler, R. C. (2000). Invisible support and adjustment to stress. *Journal of Personality and Social Psychology, 79,* 953–961.

Bowers, B. (1987). Intergenerational caregiving: Adult caregivers and their aging parents. *Advances in Nursing Science, 9,* 20–31.

Bowers, B. (1988). Family perceptions of care in a nursing home. *The Gerontologist, 28,* 361–368.

Bruce, D., & Paterson, A. (2000). Barriers to community support for the dementia carer: A qualitative study. *International Journal of Geriatric Psychiatry, 15,* 451–457.

Cantor, M. H. (1975). Life space and the social support system of the inner city elderly of New York. *The Gerontologist, 15,* 23–27.

Carpentier, N., & Ducharme, F. (2003). Caregiver network transformations: The need for an integrated perspective. *Ageing & Society, 23,* 507–525.

Chappell, N., & Blandford, A. (1991). Informal and formal care: Exploring complementarity. *Aging and Society, 11*(3), 299–317.

Clark, M. S., Mills, J., & Powell, M. C. (1986). Keeping track of needs in communal and exchange relationships. *Journal of Personality and Social Psychology, 51*(2), 333–338.

Cohen, C., Teresi, J., & Blum, C. (1994). The role of caregiver social networks in Alzheimer's disease. *Social Science & Medicine, 38*(11), 1483–1490.

Cook, K. S., & Rice, E. (2003). Social exchange theory. In J. Delamater (Ed.), *Handbook of social psychology* (pp. 53–76). New York: Kluwer Academic/Plenum.

Dunkel-Schetter, C., Folkman, S., & Lazarus, R. (1987). Correlates of social support receipt. *Journal of Personality and Social Psychology, 53,* 71–80.

Dupuis, S., & Norris, J. (1997). A multidimensional and contextual framework for understanding diverse family members' roles in long-term care facilities. *Journal of Aging Studies, 11*(4), 297–325.

Edelman, P., & Hughes, S. (1990). The impact of community care on provision of informal care to homebound elderly persons. *Journal of Gerontology: Social Sciences, 45*(Suppl.), S574–S584.

Fudge, H., Neufeld, A., & Harrison, M. H. (1997). Social networks of women caregivers. *Public Health Nursing, 14*(1), 20–27.

Goldsmith, D., & Parks, M. R. (1990). Communicative strategies for managing the risks of seeking social support. In S. Duck & R. C. Silber (Eds.), *Personal relationships and social support* (pp. 85–111). New York: Academic Press.

Harrison, M. J., & Neufeld, A. (1997). Women's experience of barriers to support while caregiving. *Health Care for Women International, 18,* 591–602.

Harrison, M. J., Neufeld, A., & Kushner, K. (1995). Women in transition: Access and barriers to social support. *Journal of Advanced Nursing, 21,* 858–864.

Hartman, A. (1995). Diagrammatic assessment of family relationships. *Families in Society: The Journal of Contemporary Human Services, 76*(2), 111–122.

Hayes, P. (2006). Home is where their health is: Rethinking perspectives of informal and formal care by older rural Appalachian women who live alone. *Qualitative Health Research, 16*(2), 282–297.

Heinrich, M., Neufeld, A., & Harrison, M. (2003). Seeking support: Caregiver strategies for interacting with health personnel. *Canadian Journal of Nursing Research, 35*(4), 38–56.

Hibbard, J., Neufeld, A., & Harrison, M. J. (1996). Gender differences in the support networks of caregivers. *Journal of Gerontological Nursing, 22*(9), 15–23.

Hochschild, A. (1989). *The second shift.* New York: Avon.

Hurst, I. (2001). Mothers' strategies to meet their needs in the newborn intensive care nursery. *Journal of Perinatal & Neonatal Nursing, 15*(2), 65–82.

Keating, N., Otfinowski, P., Wenger, C., Fast, J., & Derksen, L. (2003). Understanding the caring capacity of informal networks of frail seniors: A case for care networks. *Ageing & Society, 23*, 115–127.

Lilly, M., Richards, B., & Buckwalter, K. (2003). Friends and social support in dementia caregiving. *Journal of Gerontological Nursing, 29*(1), 29–36.

Lin, N., Dumm, M. Y., & Woelfel, M. (1986). Measuring community and network support. In N. Lin, A. Dean, & W. M. Ensel (Eds.), *Social support, life events, and depression* (pp. 153–170). London: Academic Press.

Litt, J. (2004). Women's carework in low-income households: The special case of children with attention deficit hyperactivity disorder. *Gender & Society, 18*, 625–644.

Litwak, E. (1985). *Helping the elderly: The complementary roles of informal networks and formal systems.* New York: Guilford.

Lyons, K., & Zarit, S. (1999). Formal and informal support: The great divide. *International Journal of Geriatric Psychiatry, 14*, 183–196.

Molm, L., Quist, T. M., & Wisely, P. A. (1994). Imbalanced structures, unfair strategies: Power and justice in social exchange. *American Sociological Review, 59*, 98–121.

Molm, L., Takahashi, N., & Peterson, G. (2000). Risk and trust in social exchange: An experimental test of a classical proposition. *American Journal of Sociology, 105*(5), 1396–1427.

Murray, M. (2002). Connecting narrative and social representation theory in health research. *Social Science Information, 41*(4), 653–673.

Neufeld, A., & Harrison, M. J. (1994). Men and women caregivers: Barriers to using support. In *Proceedings of the 56th Annual Conference of the National Council on Family Relations*, Minneapolis, MN. (Abstract)

Neufeld, A., & Harrison, M. J. (1995). Reciprocity and social support in caregivers' relationships: Variations and consequences. *Qualitative Health Research, 5*, 349–366.

Penning, M. J. (2002). Hydra revisited: Substituting formal for self- and informal in-home care among older adults with disabilities. *The Gerontologist, 42*(1), 4–16.

Pyke, K. D., & Bengston, V. (1996). Caring more or less: Individualistic and collectivist systems of family eldercare. *Journal of Marriage and the Family, 58*, 379–392.

Rafaeli, E., & Gleason, M. E. J. (2009). Skilled support within intimate relationships. *Journal of Family Theory & Review, 1*, 20–37.

Ray, L. D. (2002). Parenting and childhood chronicity: Making visible the invisible work. *Journal of Pediatric Nursing, 17*(6), 424–438.

Rook, K. (1990). Parallels in the study of social support and social strain. *Journal of Social and Clinical Psychology, 9*(1), 118–132.

Russell, R. (2004). Social networks among elderly men caregivers. *Journal of Men's Studies, 13*(1), 121–142.

Russell, R. (2007). Men doing "women's work": Elderly men caregivers and the gendered construction of care work. *Journal of Men's Studies, 15*, 1–18.

Sabatelli, R. M., & Shehan, C. L. (1993). Exchange and resource theories. In P. G. Boss, W. J. Doherty, R. LaRossa, W. R. Schumm, & S. K. Steinmetz (Eds.), *Sourcebook of family* (pp. 385–417). New York: Plenum.

Smith, G. C., Smith, M. F., & Toseland, R. W. (1991). Problems identified by family caregivers in counselling. *The Gerontologist, 31*, 15–22.

Thompson, L. (1991). Family work: Women's sense of fairness. *Journal of Family Issues*, *12*, 181–196.

Walker, K., MacBride, A., & Vachon, M. (1977). Social support networks and the crisis of bereavement. *Social Science & Medicine, 11*, 35–41.

Wenger, G. C. (1991). A network typology: From theory to practice. *Journal of Aging Studies, 5*(2), 147–162.

Wuest, J., Ericson, P. K., Stern, P. N., & Irwin G. W., Jr. (2001). Connected and disconnected support: The impact on caregiving support in Alzheimer's disease. *Health Care for Women International, 22*, 115–130.

Wright, L. M., & Leahey, M. (2005). *Nurses and families: A guide to family assessment and intervention* (4th ed.). Philadelphia: F. A. Davis.

5 Mobilizing Support from Professional Sources

Family caregivers receive support from formal or professional sources as well as from their informal social network of family and friends. As we indicated in Chapter 4, there are divergent perspectives on the ways in which caregivers choose to integrate assistance from professionals and from family and friends. The closeness of the relationship with potential helpers, the type of assistance required, and the extent of the caregiving demand in relation to available resources have been identified as influencing how caregivers mobilize support (Carpentier & Ducharme, 2003; Chappell & Blandford, 1991; Dupuis & Norris, 1997; Edelman & Hughes, 1990; Litwak, 1985; Penning, 2002).

Our research has addressed the personal and cultural beliefs and expectations that family caregivers hold about use of services; their perceptions of influencing factors within their network, caregiving situation, and setting; or personal skills that either facilitate (enable) or hinder (disable) the use of professional sources of support, as well as the strategies that they employ to sustain professional assistance. It is important to explore how caregivers mobilize professional sources of support, because some groups, such as men caregivers of the elderly, have been identified as not accessing services, despite a high level of need (Kaye & Applegate, 1990; Robinson, Buckwalter, & Reed, 2005; Winslow, 2003). Research with caregivers of a relative with dementia found that 64% of caregivers did not use available services and that spousal caregivers found it especially difficult to involve someone else in providing care (Robinson et al., 2005; Winslow, 2003). In addition, initial encounters with one formal resource can influence a caregiver's use of other services in relation to a variety of needs (Brown, Chen, Mitchell, & Province, 2007; Stommel, Collins, Given, & Given, 1999). A study of men caring for a wife with dementia (Brown et al., 2007) found that an initial positive experience in requesting help from community agencies or professionals increased the likelihood of using the resource again, but a negative initial experience created reluctance.

In understanding how caregivers mobilize support from both formal and informal sources, it is useful to consider their expectations and beliefs about preferred sources of support and the conditions that enable them to mobilize support within their relationships (Badr, Acitelli, Duck, & Carl, 2001). In this chapter, we illustrate the perceptions of caregivers, and the strategies they used to mobilize and maintain access to professional sources of support, by discussing our research on the experience of men and women caring for a relative with dementia. We begin by describing the process that men caregivers experienced in confronting their need for assistance and ultimately seeking placement for their relative with dementia in a long-term care facility. We next discuss the strategies women used in interaction with professionals in community agencies, particularly staff in long-term care facilities.

MEN CAREGIVERS

Confronting the Need for Assistance: Making Concessions for Care

In a study of men caregivers of a relative with dementia, most of whom were spouses, we found that men were very reluctant to disclose the challenges they had and to accept assistance with their caregiving (Coe & Neufeld, 1999). For as long as possible, the men preferred to give care to their spouse by themselves or with the help of family and friends. When these sources became insufficient to meet the caregiving demands, the men reluctantly yielded to the involvement of professional help. During the course of using professional help from health or social service agencies, the men struggled to make decisions that allowed them to maintain their own values and beliefs, provide for the well-being of the care recipient, and maintain their own physical and emotional health. In an effort to achieve this balance, however, men caregivers often had to modify their beliefs and personal expectations about the recipient's care or change their health practices.

We labeled the central phenomenon that men experienced in relation to mobilizing support from professionals "making concessions for care." The caregivers experienced the process of making concessions for care in four sequential phases: resisting, giving in, opening the door, and making the match. Although the men maintained their opposition to the involvement of formal help during the phase of resisting, they recognized the need during the phase of giving in. Men caregivers made contact with a professional source of help in the phase of opening the door. Finally, making the match involved the process of continually finding suitable sources of help to meet changing needs. Influences on the process of securing assistance included characteristics—of both the health care system and individual staff members—that had facilitating or hindering effects. For caregivers whose use of formal support included the admission of their relative to a long-term facility, the phase of making the match was followed by redesigning their caregiving role. The men differed in their response to use of formal support once a source of assistance had been accessed.

Phase 1: Resisting

The personal beliefs and expectations of the men caregivers prevented them from seeking help with care. The most common reasons for resisting support from health and social agencies were a desire to maintain independence, a sense of personal responsibility for caregiving, and personal pride. Three men expressed their view in the examples that follow.

> If it's got to get done, I'll just do it myself. I don't go around looking for help.

> I always figure that was my responsibility, nobody else's.

> I can't ask for help . . . it's just not my character. . . . I'm a very proud man . . . even applying for home care was difficult for me.

Other reasons for resisting help from community agencies with the care of their relative were perceived difficulty or dishonor in seeking help from social agencies outside the family, a strong value on family privacy, and the perceived obligation to do something in return for any assistance received.

> You look after yourself and you look after your own family, and it's a sin—no, not a sin, but it's a sort of a dishonor or something or other to seek help from social agencies. We have been brought up to keep things within the home . . . what goes on between Dad and Mom is nobody's business but our own.

Another caregiver described his perspective this way:

> If somebody does help me, I must give them something, a remuneration of some kind. . . . I insist on it so, I feel that I do owe that.

Other feelings that influenced the mobilization of support included embarrassment about the diagnosis of Alzheimer's disease and anxiety related to their inexperience in asking for help. One caregiver, who did not resist seeking professional help, had learned, from his experience with an Alcoholics Anonymous group, how to help and be helped by others.

Phase 2: Giving In

In the second phase, giving in, caregivers had to overcome personal help-seeking barriers and request support. One male caregiver identified how he overcame his reluctance to seek help from a social agency. He found it more acceptable to access that help through the physician.

> I suppose now we've had Medicare long enough that we're getting used to socialized medicine . . . and we don't have the stigma attached there any more to seeking help. And that was my approach, through the doctor, because I was getting to the end of my rope.

Acknowledgment of the need for formal help was preceded by a critical experience, a specific event, or a series of behaviors by the care recipient that caused the caregiving demands to exceed the caregiver's emotional or physical ability.

I woke up one time, and he was in my room with a screwdriver . . . just hovering above my face with a screwdriver. I don't know if he would have hurt me, but it was this . . . very unpredictable [behavior] that kind of brought it to a [head]. I took him to see [the doctor], and that same day he was taken over to [an institution].

Another man commented,

I got to the point where I just said to her, "Doctor, look, I need some help. I can't keep this up."

Phase 3: Opening the Door

When caregivers actually sought help from agencies or professionals, they entered the next phase, opening the door. Although they were now ready to accept help, they encountered other barriers, such as a lack of information and not knowing where to go for help.

The average individual is not aware of what's out there until he gets involved in it and starts getting some of the feedback. But to start with, he hasn't got a clue where to start.

The key to opening the door for caregivers was contact with a link, usually a health professional or a representative of the Alzheimer's Society, who provided information about care options and, in some cases, facilitated access to care. In each case, the process of opening the door was initiated by the caregiver, unless a critical experience resulted in hospitalization of their relative:

There is help there if you just go after it. The help doesn't find you. You have to go after the help.

Caregivers also encountered other obstacles once such a link was found—for example, if there was a delay in obtaining assistance, policies restricted the assistance that could be provided, or the application process was long and complex.

The nurse from the day hospital . . . thought we'd get started before Christmas. Well we didn't, it was January before they started her in over there. So I had another 3 months all on my own.

Another male caregiver talks about the delay and lack of assistance.

> All this time I was looking after her at home and also trying to get her into a care home and it seemed like, as though, there was never a place for her to go.

Opening the door to help from agencies or professionals through the referral process was separate from hiring supplementary help. Some caregivers whose annual income exceeded a low income level (> $20,000 CDN) chose to hire help to supplement the care they gave at home and the care their relative received in community facilities. The caregivers exercised complete control in the hiring process, and some caregivers viewed it as a business arrangement.

> Anything else I wanted in the way of help, um, I went out and purchased . . . I went out as I was running, just like I'm running a business and I need it, I went out and bought it, like nursing help, care dropping in, and this sort of thing.

Phase 4: Making the Match

Once the men found a professional who could acquaint them with care options, they entered into a process of matching services from the formal system with their needs and those of the recipient. The two processes involved in making the match were *engaging formal help* and, when the care recipient was admitted to a long-term care facility, *redesigning the caregiver role.*

In engaging formal help, the caregivers acknowledged their needs, selected from among the options available in their community, used an option, and evaluated its effectiveness. The process was ongoing and circular; the caregivers continued to acknowledge needs as they occurred and to select or decline other care options.

> I think that was a good part of the difficulty with that program . . . we had mismatched the patient and the program . . . having found that it was a mismatch, ah, I got assistance in finding a better matchup.

Although caregivers sought formal assistance in maintaining care for their relative in the home, one of the most challenging decisions was admitting the care recipient to a long-term care facility. The caregivers struggled with the option to use institutional care and resisted it for as long as possible.

> I wouldn't want to put her in there as long as I can look after her. As long as I can do it, I'm going to do it for her.

Another man described his experience in not using long-term care when it became available:

> I had her on a waiting list to go into the [nursing home], but the time came to it, and I couldn't find it in my heart to put her in there.

Despite the use of community resources, often a critical experience occurred that preceded acknowledgment of the need for institutional care. When selecting institutional care, the caregiver went through a process of convincing himself and giving over. Convincing himself involved deciding that institutional care was best. Sometimes this process continued long after the recipient was placed in institutional care.

> I'll keep telling myself, well look, they're looking after her better than what you can, and convincing myself of that, and I think it will work out.

Another male caregiver said,

> I spent every day at the hospital until I run myself ragged, and they kept telling me, but of course I wouldn't listen. Now I tell others [that taking a break is important].

Giving over was the actual act of relinquishing care to the institution and was difficult for the men.

> I just had [it]; as sad as it was, I just couldn't do any more myself.

Another man talks about his feelings when his wife entered long-term care:

> I have every Tuesday . . . the chaplain closes the door and then we start, and the tears flow like wine . . . this is the only place I can really relieve my tension.

Although most caregivers first accepted community-based help, a few used long-term care almost immediately. The element of safety and the level of care required by the care recipient were the distinguishing features. Caregivers who faced safety issues and whose loved one required a high of personal care did not go through the process of selecting other community options before placement in long-term care.

Factors Influencing Men's Experience in Securing Professional Support

Throughout the process of making the match, men caregivers were influenced by the behavior of professionals and by characteristics of the health care system. Facilitating behaviors of professionals were those that directly assisted the men in dealing with their caregiving situation or indirectly assisted them by enhancing the well-being of their spouse, the care recipient. These facilitating behaviors included comforting the caregivers, demonstrating a caring attitude toward the men and their spouses, addressing problems associated with the care recipient, affirming the role the men had assumed, providing assistance with caregiving tasks, and providing information.

> There's one social worker, she's extremely good with me, and we go out every couple of weeks for lunch . . . we can sit and talk about anything to each other, and that's been most helpful.

Another man described how helpful respite care was.

> That was the first time we ever used it [respite], so it was with quite some trepidation that I left her in the care of others for the very first time. . . . I can't speak highly enough of how well they looked after her . . . made me feel really good.

In contrast, the caregivers perceived some behaviors of professionals that hindered their ability to access aid from professional sources. Such behaviors detracted from the caregiver's role or interfered with meeting the care recipient's needs. These behaviors included inadequate communication with caregivers, exclusion of the men from involvement in decisions about the care recipient, exclusion of the men caregivers from providing care to their relative, provision of advice that the men perceived as detrimental to the care recipient, and behavior that showed a lack of understanding toward the caregiver or the care recipient.

> And I can't talk to doctors because they just have 15 minutes or if you're lucky they give you half an hour. . . . I can't even remember the numbers of things that I want to talk about.

One man described his experience in this way:

> We get into scraps . . . mainly because they [the staff in long-term care] do things and they don't stop to think what effect it's going to have on anybody but themselves . . . who's making all these decisions that all of a sudden we're encouraged to do one thing and they tell us they're going to do another thing? What's going on here?

For another caregiver, establishing what care he could give was challenging:

> I'm even limited now [with] how much I can help him in an institution, how much they're willing to let me do. I don't think they want me to do it [bathing the care recipient] on my own, and I don't know if they even want me to do it, period.

The men also described characteristics of the system that hindered their access to services, including a lack of coordination in the care placement process, policies that restricted the provision of service, a lack of appropriate facilities to manage the care recipient's aggressive behavior, inadequate assessment of the recipient, inadequate staffing, inadequate standards of care, and cost.

> We went from [one lodge] to a nursing home . . . to another nursing home . . . [then] they punch you into one that you haven't chosen because it's available, and then . . . the one you selected is now available so now you move across there . . . it took . . . 6 months [for the care recipient] to remember which door was his where he was living for a year, and to constantly move . . . it's a real pain.

In some cases, the service available was not really what the caregiver required.

> I really didn't need the housework done so much as I wanted time off . . . I'd ask them to take [the care recipient] for a walk . . . for a while they objected to that because . . . their bosses figured that they should be cleaning house.

In other situations, the service available to the care recipient was not well matched.

> He does not belong in a mental hospital. He belongs in a care home that can handle aggressive behavior, which we don't have in this country.

Another caregiver experienced the consequences of an inaccurate assessment that was responsible for an inappropriate placement.

> The nurse that assessed her had assessed her wrong . . . out of desperation the head nurse phoned me and said . . . "The form said she wasn't incontinent" . . . she sounded so desperate I went and brought [the care recipient] out again.

Cost is often an influence on resources accessed, and caregivers varied in their views on the cost of care. Some felt the cost was reasonable, but others felt it was too high.

Consequences of the Use of Support Services

The men caregivers' response to their use of support from agencies and professionals included their feelings about the process of securing and using the help, their perception of the value of the help, and their ability to create a new life after the care recipient entered a long-term care facility. These responses further influenced how they engaged formal help. Caregivers were most often concerned about the adequacy of care for the recipient and expressed both positive and negative assessments of the care their relative received.

> [The nurses] are phenomenal . . . I don't know how they do their job, they're great.

Conflict in the caregivers' relationships with staff resulted in anger and frustration. The most common focus of the conflict was the caregivers' concerns about the well-being of their relatives and the adequacy of the care provided.

> There must be better care than what I've seen or witnessed at times. It's hard to see people strapped in chairs.

Those caregivers who experienced conflict with agency personnel and professionals experienced added stress.

> It is bad enough going through the experience with a person you care about, but to have to fight uphill with everybody to get him to the place where he should be was extremely tiring.

Men caregivers also expressed both positive and negative feelings about their experiences as caregivers in seeking support. Some described feelings of frustration, helplessness, uncertainty, displeasure, desperation, and shame.

> At home it was most difficult until we finally broke the ice . . . it must be frustrating for a lot of other people . . . when you call an agency that should be able to help you and they say, "No, we can't."

Other men recognized the value of help from professionals and agencies in getting their needs met, as well as meeting the needs of the care recipient. Assistance from these sources could increase their understanding of the system and improve the men's health.

> This last week I haven't felt anywhere near as tense . . . accepting that [the care recipient] is in where she's being properly cared for [in long-term care]. . . . I don't have to sit here and worry . . . the result of this is my stomach has been fine . . . and I seem to be sleeping far better.

Caregivers who placed their relative in a long-term care facility gradually created a new life for themselves, while maintaining a commitment to their loved ones. A new life was manifested by increased social and recreational activity. The caregivers that we interviewed were in different stages of accomplishing this process, as the following quotations from two men illustrate:

I don't know how you handle this "You should wash your hands and start your life over again" type of thing. I guess it's hard for me.

Another man said,

I've realized that she's there being attended, the best of care that is available. I have a life to live, so get on and start living and don't sulk. . . . Meet people, do things . . . I'm coming out.

Men caregivers were confronted with the challenge of learning new ways of caring for their relatives once they were admitted to a long-term care setting. Because they no longer retained sole responsibility for their relative, they redesigned their caregiving role to provide care for the care recipient while they shared their expert knowledge of their relative's health issues and need for care with professionals. They also expanded their role by helping other family caregivers and care recipients.

A consequence of admitting their relative to long-term care was the challenge of redesigning their caregiving role. Men continued to provide care, primarily through activities related to feeding, walking, and taking the recipient on outings. They provided stimulation through activities, such as reading the newspaper aloud to the recipient, and maintained the recipient's personal identity, by celebrating events such as birthdays or buying favorite foods. A few caregivers were not as involved in providing care, but they continued to visit. The frequency and duration of visits varied among caregivers. In providing care, the caregivers were sensitive to a boundary between their role and that of professionals. The men were cautious not to overstep what they perceived to be the domain of the staff, yet they wanted to retain involvement in care. Caregivers shared their expert knowledge of the care recipient with professionals.

I don't know anyone who knows my wife's condition or any little idiosyncrasies that she has better than myself because we've been married 47 years, and the doctor, who sees her once a month for 5 minutes and is out the door, knows very little about her.

Men expanded their caregiving role by helping other caregivers and care recipients. They used a variety of metaphors (e.g., "same boat," "same shoes," "I've kind of been down the road. . . . I can give some good direction") to describe their ability to relate to other caregivers.

I see these new patients come in. I see their families coming in, and I do not hesitate to go up, shake hands with them, introduce myself, and put an arm around them and tell them I know where they're coming from and how they're feeling.

They comforted other caregivers directly through individual contact, sharing their experiences at informal meetings and support groups, representing caregivers on committees, writing about their experiences, and educating the public about Alzheimer's disease. They also helped meet the needs of other patients and advocated on their behalf.

In the next section, we describe our study of women caring for a relative with dementia, as another illustration of the perspective and experience of family caregivers in mobilizing support from professionals and health and social agencies. In this study, we focused on the strategies that women family caregivers employed in interactions with health personnel from community agencies, such as home care and long-term care services. We examined how women caregivers sought to sustain support through use of these interaction strategies (Heinrich, Neufeld, & Harrison, 2003).

WOMEN CAREGIVERS

Strategies in Interactions with Health Personnel

Once a linkage was established with an agency or professional, women caregivers used varied strategies—*collaborating, getting along, twigging, fighting*—to sustain assistance from professional sources. Their use of these strategies varied according to their perception of the degree of mutuality or collaboration between themselves and professionals in decision making. Although we describe the strategies individually, each caregiver might use several strategies simultaneously in her interactions with personnel. The women's perception of the caregiving experience varied according to the strategies that were used. For example, when women caregivers were able to collaborate with professionals in providing care to their family members, a process that entailed a high degree of mutuality, they perceived their caregiving experience as positive. When they fought or struggled with staff of an agency over the care that was provided, on the other hand, mutuality was absent, and the women care-

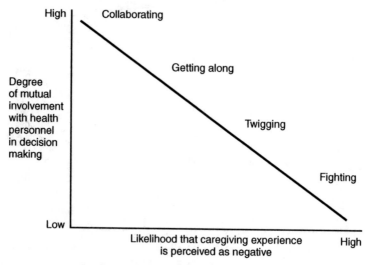

Figure 5.1. Interactional strategies in relation to the perception of caregiving experience and mutual involvement with health personnel.

givers perceived their experience as negative. These strategies and the caregivers' experiences are illustrated in Figure 5.1.

Collaborating

Collaborating occurred when the caregiver's relationship with agency staff was characterized by the sharing of information and goals. In these complementary relationships, the caregivers contributed their knowledge of their family member and previously successful care strategies to the decision-making process of how their family member would receive care. In turn, the staff in long-term care provided information on services and suggested alternative care approaches. They also valued the contribution of the family caregiver. One woman described this collaboration.

> We get our heads together with [the] charge nurse . . . Any time we have a problem, we all get our heads together and deal with it.

Another woman described the staff's sharing of information at a conference soon after her family member had been placed in a nursing home:

I think one of the things that I really found helpful was . . . a caregivers' conference . . . I learned more from that and felt more at home, more able to relate to those people, [I] better understood what they did and why they did it.

The opportunity for collaboration was facilitated by certain characteristics of the caregiver's relationship with health personnel. Some professionals affirmed the women's caregiving work by praising the caring work that they had done; others expressed emotional support for the woman caregiver. For example, a physician affirmed the woman's caregiving role:

He [the physician] said, "You look after your mother, but you don't let her sit around and vegetate." . . . He knew how I always kept her going . . . there were always some little chores for her to do.

Staff members expressed their emotional support by taking an interest in both the caregiver and the care recipient, being friendly, having a positive attitude, and showing compassion.

When I see them [the home care nurse and the physician], they always ask . . . . People don't realize how much that helps . . . just asking, "Is there anything I can [do]?" or "How are things going?" . . . Then you know they care . . . they wouldn't ask, otherwise.

Other professionals or agency staff demonstrated an understanding of family caregiving that was based in personal experience as well as professional knowledge. The women valued interactions in which a staff member who had personal family caregiving experience shared this experience with them. They believed that only those personnel who understood the caregiver and their relative with dementia could provide the affirmation and emotional support necessary to facilitate collaboration. Such understanding required both formal education and practical experience in caring for an elderly person with dementia.

Collaborating was inhibited, however, when caregivers were excluded from decision making. They often attributed their exclusion to inadequate knowledge and lack of understanding on the part of staff. Some women caregivers said that the care needs of their relative were not being met because staff had inadequate knowledge. One woman was frustrated and angry when she learned, incidentally, that her mother had long been receiving an anti-anxiety agent without her knowledge.

> She was like a zombie. . . . It was bothering me terribly. . . . I called the doctor. . . . The nurse . . . said, "Oh . . . I think your mother should be cut back on the tranquilizers," and I said, "The what?" And I found out at this time that they had her on . . . Ativan three times a day. . . . This is what her problem [was]. . . . Then I was really angry.

Stereotyping by health personnel was another barrier to collaborating.

> They're inclined maybe to stereotype people . . . especially a younger [staff member]. I mean, a hundred [years old]—you're supposed to be out for the count . . . [but] we knew different.

The women felt that stereotyping encouraged a standardized rather than an individualized approach to care. Some women also thought that illness in elderly people was treated less seriously than in young people.

> It was really scary how weak she was, and . . . listles . . . They were saying they were feeding her . . . Nobody saw it. . . . She was just weaker and weaker, and they were accommodating her weakness by keeping her in bed and feeding her and doing nothing about it.

This woman felt that staff overlooked her mother's symptoms because they attributed the changes to the aging process rather than to a specific health issue.

When caregivers were able to collaborate with staff, they expressed satisfaction with their relationships with health care providers. Collaboration served to affirm their contribution to the care of their relative and increase their understanding of the role and contribution of health care providers. When women were able to engage in collaboration with professionals, they perceived the caregiving experience as positive.

Getting Along

Sometimes the women used a strategy of getting along to establish and maintain a good working relationship with personnel in institutional and home care settings. In adopting this strategy, the women were not yet engaged in a negotiated relationship with staff, but they had assumed personal responsibility for maintaining a positive connection, despite indifference or intimidation on the part of staff. They viewed staff members as busy and tired and were reluctant to be a "pest." One woman said it was not easy to talk to staff members "standing there in a uniform . . . in a hurry and [with] things on their minds." They reported that personnel responded abruptly to their requests for information, were threatened by their questions, or viewed the caregiver as snooping or checking up on them. The women felt that staff members were less available to them as a source of support if the staff member was very young or, because of frequent staff turnover, was a stranger.

Getting along had two components: initiating action diplomatically and negotiating among multiple providers. One woman described how she initiated action diplomatically when she found something amiss with the care recipient:

> I get things going . . . I don't go [to the nursing home] . . . half-cocked, either, because I'm annoyed . . . [I say,] "Let's just see what the problem is."

A woman caring for her husband at home had to negotiate among multiple health professionals and secure their ongoing commitment. This was demanding and stressful work.

> A lot of your time is spent just acting as a little go-between . . . and hoping everybody will get along . . . to buoy everybody up . . . to keep going for [the care recipient] and be cheerful and keep Home Care going, and always negotiating, always having to . . . play the end against the middle and hope somebody won't get angry or quit or [that] this won't fall apart.

The primary factors influencing the use of the strategy of getting along were perceived discomfort, intimidation, or indifference in relationships with agency staff. Getting along enabled the women to maintain a satisfactory relationship with professional but it inhibited the free exchange of information. For example, one woman expressed overall satisfaction with her interactions with formal providers but said that caregivers sometimes withheld information from staff because they were afraid of the response.

> We don't always tell [health personnel] everything we'd like to tell them. They're just not another shoulder to cry on . . . they're paid to do their job . . . . Lots of times we're afraid to tell them some of the things we'd like to.

The women also found getting along to be fatiguing:

> You're just giving like that all the time, and that's very tiring.

The women who employed this strategy often found their caregiving role to be a negative one. Getting along made them feel that they were doing all of the relationship work. Their relationship with health personnel could be characterized as draining.

Twigging

Some women described "twigging" the staff to unmet needs, or showing them how to meet the needs of the care recipient. The caregivers also shared information about changes in the health status of their family member. Although some women felt this was part of their caregiving role, because it was they who best knew the care recipient, other caregivers were disappointed by the inattention of the staff.

One woman tried daily to have nursing home personnel insert her mother's dentures and hearing aid, which, she said, were important for her mother's quality of life, even though she could not ask for them herself. The daughter was frustrated that these basics were being neglected, even though she had posted signs to remind staff. Another woman was concerned about her mother's declining appetite. She was disappointed that she had to ask nursing home staff to give her mother a dietary supplement. Another woman had to speak up to ensure that her husband was included in social activities at the nursing home.

Twigging included teaching others, including health personnel, how to be helpful. One woman spent a great deal of time teaching the care attendants who came to her home how to meet the complex care needs of her husband. Women initiated twigging or sharing of information when their vigilance revealed inadequacies in care or a change in their relative's health status that put them at risk. Use of this strategy implied that the women expected staff to act on their feedback. The women found that twigging could be stressful.

It kind of concerned me that any time I made a big fuss about something or other they would retaliate on my mom . . . . When her glasses disappeared at one time, I [wondered], did they take them away from her . . . because I had complained about something?

As the prior quotation illustrates, some women were unable to establish a comfortable, collaborative relationship with staff in planning care, and they feared retaliation from the staff against the care recipient if they consistently urged health personnel to change their relative's care.

Fighting

Several women described their interactions with health personnel in institutional or home settings using words such as "fighting" or "battle." Unlike twigging, which was intended to elicit a positive response from staff, this strategy was employed when staff did not readily respond to caregivers' information about their relative and they believed their relative was at risk. Their stories indicated that they were prepared to act until they secured the help needed.

One woman planned to persevere until she obtained information about the medications administered to her mother, who resided in a nursing home. In the past, this woman had received a monthly itemized list of her mother's medications and dosages. When her mother was reassessed at a higher level of care, she no longer received this information because the government paid for the medications:

I'm not getting an itemized list from them. . . . They will give the normal printout of the drugs the doctor orders . . . but not the specific amount in a month that is actually administered to her, which is what I want . . . I will not let it rest. There will be some way . . . maybe I'll have to go as far as being declared a legal guardian . . . which I will do.

One caregiver was frustrated when she had to wait for necessary equipment for her home before her husband could be discharged from hospital:

It went back and forth . . . I had to change the whole back entry . . . because he couldn't [climb] stairs. . . . We put a lift in. . . . They told me there's a grant for people like that. So I applied for the grant, and I was pushed on time because [the hospital] had to discharge him. . . . I was on the phone every day. . . . I said, "I need this, and I need this." So I was between the [hospital], who would like to send him home, and Home Care, who had the red tape from here to Rome.

Another woman had to fight to secure adequate personal care for her family member:

I have battled it out with Home Care . . . I have worked very hard on that . . . . I do qualify for the time, and I did get it . . . [but] with the Home Care situation you have to remember that it is re-evaluated very frequently, and at any moment you may be cut back or you might have to go to bat for what you've got in the . . . first place.

She went on to describe the advice she would give to other caregivers:

You have to be prepared for a long, long wait with the services . . . applications for pensions, you're looking at a year to a year and a half . . . it goes on forever; you just have to keep on going. . . . If you want something, just don't back off. I mean, if you keep at it long enough . . . they're going to say yes to get rid of you.

The women used the fighting strategy when their attempts to obtain support were met by a long wait, when their initial requests for help were rejected, or when they had to appeal a decision about the amount of support allocated. These experiences were highly stressful.

Women employing this strategy lacked affirmation in their caregiving role and were frustrated by their inability to secure the assistance their relative needed. Although they found it stressful, they considered this strategy a necessary part of caregiving if the health of their relative was threatened. They felt it was the only way they could ensure a satisfactory level of care.

Factors Influencing Women Caregivers' Interactions with Health Personnel

The women caregivers used the preceding strategies to secure and sustain assistance with their caregiving role as well as assistance for their relative, which indirectly relieved their perceived demands as a caregiver. In seeking support, the women interacted with health personnel on behalf of their relative. These actions required the women to maintain a constant vigil, monitoring the care recipient and seeking information from all available sources.

The women's expectations of themselves as family caregivers and their assessment of their relative influenced their work as caregivers and their strategies in interacting with health personnel. For example, they described a keen sense of personal responsibility and a belief that they were the best persons to take care of their relatives:

> I'm the only one around who is really close to my mom, that knows her . . . What if I was in that same position and I didn't have anyone around that really . . . cared about me . . . knew the way I used to be?

Women who were daughters, daughters-in-law, or granddaughters considered caregiving an opportunity to reciprocate for all the elder's past contributions. The wives spoke of a strong marriage commitment, believing their husband would do the same for them. When the marital relationship was conflicted, they described their caregiving role as an obligation. Family expectations also supported the women's belief in filial responsibility.

> My mom kept saying, "We never put our people in a nursing home" . . . . That was a very powerful message to me.

One woman feared she would be disowned by her family if she did not continue to care for her husband on her own.

> I think I'll go over and say to them, "Are you going to disown me if I put him in long-term care?"

Because of personal and family beliefs that women are responsible for caregiving and are the "best" caregivers, the participants were vulnerable to a sense of failure when they sought assistance. They continued to view themselves as responsible for care of their relative. The perceived expectations of health personnel and health care policies also influenced their interactions with personnel and their requests for help. For example, one woman described a need to establish a good track record; she felt she had to demonstrate that she had done everything she could before the professionals would consider her request for help. Others thought that nursing home staff expected them to do more for their relative, and the wives believed that physicians expected them to be there for their husbands. Nearly all of the women believed that health care resources are scarce and accepted the societal expectation that public resources should be available only to those who need them most. This made them hesitant to seek help. In some cases, the women waited until a crisis occurred before requesting aid.

Assessment of their relative's cognitive status influenced the caregivers' ability to secure assistance. However, the unpredictability of the course of dementia made it difficult for them to anticipate when they would need help. The women did not want to place their relative in a nursing home before it was necessary, but they found it difficult to know when to make the decision, particularly because facilities had waiting lists with uncertain wait times. As a result of the variation and unpredictability of the care recipient's cognitive status, it was difficult for the women to get timely and appropriate assistance.

When the care recipient was in the early stages of dementia, the women could access help from formal sources only when it was acceptable to their relative. One woman described talking the care recipient into accepting certain kinds of help, but the mother of another woman refused to sign the necessary forms because she did not want to have people in her home.

> In order to really get my mother [into] the system, she would have to sign the forms, which of course she would refuse to do because she doesn't need any help in her mind—"Thank you very much, but get out of here."

This caregiver did not want to go against her mother's wishes and seek guardianship through the courts. In the later stages of caregiving, however, it became easier for her to access help, because the care recipient was unaware of what was happening. At this stage in the dementia, the women caregivers felt they were able to make decisions on behalf of their family member.

DISCUSSION

We begin our discussion with reflection on the caregivers' desire for mutuality in their interactions with professionals in the context of the theoretical perspective of exchange theory. Relationships with professionals differ from those with members of the informal social network, such as family and friends. Interactions with professionals may more closely fit the concept of negotiated exchanges than the concept of reciprocal exchanges, which are more typical of interactions with family and friends. We conclude with a discussion of the process of mobilizing resources from the informal and formal social networks in relation to other research and perspectives on the intersection of the informal and formal support networks as sources of support for caregivers.

The importance of mutuality in interactions with professionals, as found in our research with caregivers of a relative with dementia, is also evident in research and theoretical models of the relationship between health personnel and family caregivers of persons who do not have a diagnosis of dementia (Eales, Keating, & Damsma, 2001; Gladstone & Wexler, 2002; Guberman & Maheu, 2002; Ward-Griffin & McKeever, 2000) and who receive either home care (Guberman & Maheu, 2002; Ward-Griffin & McKeever, 2000) or long-term care (Gladstone & Wexler, 2002). The theme implicit in these models of the caregiver-professional relationship is a desire for mutuality with staff, concerning decisions about care, and negative outcomes when mutuality is not achieved.

Family caregivers' emphasis on mutuality with professionals in making decisions about care for their relative confirms similar findings in two other Canadian studies in long-term care (Gladstone & Wexler, 2002; Legault & Ducharme, 2009). Gladstone and Wexler (2002) generated a model of five types of family-staff relationships: collegial, professional, friendship, distant, and tense. Collegial, professional, and friendship relationships involved interactions with staff that were focused around a specific purpose, shared experiences, and a sense of trust. They were accompanied by positive feelings. Similar to the strategy of fighting identified in our findings, Gladstone and Wexler found that distant or tense relationships emerged when family caregivers were critical or distrustful of staff, angry, or frustrated. Legault and Ducharme (2009) interviewed daughters of elders with dementia and identified collaboration and reciprocity with staff in long-term care as important strategies used by the daughters when their parent was admitted to a long-term care facility. Although their study was not specifically framed within an exchange perspective, Legault and Ducharme used the term *reciprocity* to describe an exchange of information, in which the daughter received regular information from the staff about the health and needs of her parent. In turn, the daughter had an opportunity to share her own knowledge and expertise as a family caregiver with the staff. They also report the importance of communication strategies used by the family caregiver to maintain the collaboration, citing a diplomatic communication style very similar to our strategies of *getting along* and *twigging*.

A systematic review of studies that examined staff-family relationships in the care of older people (Haesler, Bauer, & Nay, 2007) reported a variety of evidence that families of older adults in care often adopt a monitoring role to ensure that their relative receives personalized care of a satisfactory quality. Family members used strategies similar to those we report to maintain the level of control they wanted over their relative's care.

Professionals' negative expectations hindered mutuality and the ability of family caregivers in our research to seek assistance, and this information confirms the findings of other researchers. For example, expectations of staff and the psychological environment of the care unit influenced the ability of family caregivers of relatives with Alzheimer's disease to reach consensus with staff (Hurley, Volicer, Rempusheski, & Fry, 1995). In a psychiatric hospital in the United Kingdom, family caregivers were dissatisfied because professional agendas dominated meetings with staff, there was no follow-up, they felt excluded, they lacked information about how decisions were made, staff were not proactive in approaching them, and caregivers were reluctant to disturb them (Walker & Jane Dewar, 2001). In a Swedish study, Hertzberg and Ekman (2000) reported that staff thought family caregivers had unrealistic expectations and that family caregivers were frustrated by a lack of staff follow-up on their inquiries and were distrustful of staff members, despite viewing them as "nice." Staff and family caregivers did not let one another know what they were thinking. The authors commented that each group appeared to avoid learning whether their view of the other was accurate. On the other hand, caregivers were satisfied with their participation in decision making when information was shared, caregivers were included in decisions, there was a person available to contact, and the service agency was responsive to their needs (Walker & Jane Dewar, 2001). A systematic review identified that interventions designed to promote constructive family relationships were more likely to be effective if the focus of the intervention was strengthening collaboration between staff and family members (Haesler et al., 2007).

The emphasis of caregivers on mutuality in relationships with professionals may also be considered in the context of two forms of support that have been identified in research on interventions and support of families. This research suggests a distinction between supportive approaches that engage the autonomy of support recipients, labeled nondirective support, and those that do not, labeled directive support (Fisher, 1997; Fisher, LaGreca, Greco, Arfken, & Schneiderman, 1997;

Harber, Schneider, Everard, & Fisher, 2005). Directive and nondirective support are discussed in relation to professional interventions as well as support from family and friends. The primary distinction is whether the manner in which support is offered takes into account the autonomy and preferences of the support recipient (Rafaeli & Gleason, 2009). The findings of this research may help explain the reason for the ineffectiveness of intended support that does not match the expectations of the recipient for the manner of delivery, despite addressing an area of need.

The mutuality with professionals that family caregivers in our research described involved interactions in which the agency and institutional staff shared power in decision making with the family caregiver. When mutuality was not present, the caregiver felt compelled to use other strategies to get input into decisions.

The perspective of negotiated exchanges (Cook & Emerson, 1978; Cook & Rice, 2003; Molm, Peterson, & Takahashi, 1999; Molm, Quist, & Wisely, 1994) may help explain our findings on the importance of mutuality in interactions with professionals, because caregivers sought resources, such as hours of home care, from professionals who had the power to decide whether the family caregiver met the requirements of the agency. The hesitance of some caregivers to seek services could relate to their reluctance to enter into a negotiated exchange in which professionals hold more power. The costs of loss of control over the care of their relative and possible loss of family approval, for example on admitting a relative to long-term care, may be higher than the anticipated rewards. From this theoretical perspective, caregivers may have delayed accessing professional services until a crisis occurred in their own health or in the care requirements of their relative. Once their family member was admitted to a program or care facility, the use of indirect methods to obtain support, such as twigging, may also reflect the caregiver's concern over a lack of power in negotiations with professionals and agency staff. When health care workers chose a mutual form of interaction, in which they acknowledged the caregiver's skill in providing care, they reduced the power imbalance. Repeated mutual interactions between family caregivers and professionals build trust and might contribute to the perception of caregivers that relationships are collaborative and enable them to seek support.

Caregivers in our research experienced a complex process of making concessions for care as they confronted the need for assistance, either within the home or from community resources. Several phases in the process of making concessions for care are similar to the processes identified in other qualitative studies of caregivers prior to admission of their relative with dementia to a long-term care facility. For example, other researchers have described the experience of family caregivers as "surviving on the brink," in which all the alternatives available to the caregiver were undesirable (Wilson, 1989); a "fatalistic career," in which caregivers endured demands and then exited caregiving with their relative's admission to long-term care (Lindgren, 1993); "being in control," in which caregivers sought control over caregiving that was then relinquished with their relative's admission (Willoughby & Keating, 1991); or "becoming strangers," which involved a process of dawning, holding on, and relinquishing care (Wuest, Ericson, & Stern, 1994). In our findings and those of others (Dellasega & Mastrian, 1995), caregiving continued after the care recipient was admitted to long-term care but was redefined.

The importance of fit between a caregiver's beliefs and need for support and the services available has been identified in a number of studies. Men in our research who were caring for a relative with dementia and sought professional assistance were influenced by beliefs about the importance of privacy, independence, and personal responsibility, as well as assessment of their personal situation, when they sought a professional resource that fit their needs. A framework specific for community service use among caregivers of persons with Alzheimer's disease identified similar factors as influential for a caregiver's use of services (Collins, King, Given, & Given, 1994). The concept of fit, or lack of fit, between what was required and what was available was also identified in a qualitative study of Appalachian women. Hayes (2006) found that women's perception of a lack of fit with available services was often related to personal values and practices and argued that cultural beliefs and preferred ways of living are often not considered when professionals assess service options, which could result in failure of the caregiver to use available services. Values of independence and responsibility, as well as culturally specific values, played an important role in participants' ability to access and benefit from community services.

Further evidence of the importance of fit for effective support is research on social support within couple relationships, which has addressed matching of support with the coping needs of recipients on multiple dimensions (Rafaeli & Gleason, 2009). For example, some research on perceived need for support found that a greater fit between what was desired and what was provided was associated with better marital adjustment and quality (Dehle, Larsen, & Landers, 2001).

In mobilizing support from professional sources, caregivers in our research engaged in a complex help-seeking process. From their perspective, an integration of support from both family or friends and professional sources was needed to sustain caregiving. Their experience of interactions with professional sources of support was influenced by values and beliefs that are often overlooked in professional decisions. For caregivers, the concept of fit—between what they required and what was available—and the concept of mutuality in interactions with professionals were key attributes of support from professional sources.

As indicated in our introduction to Chapter 4, caregivers rely on support from both informal and formal support networks. Several divergent models of the ways in which professional and kin/friend sources of support intersect within family caregiving situations have been proposed, often with limited research support (Dupuis & Norris, 1997; Penning, 2002). There is increasing acknowledgment, however, of the strength of an integrative perspective in understanding the intersection of resources in family caregiving (Carpentier & Ducharme, 2003; Lyons & Zarit, 1999; Sebern, 2005). For example, there is evidence that family caregivers play an important role in the care of a relative in residential settings, that the relationship and intersection of roles between family and professional caregivers is a complex pattern that changes over time, and that the relationship between family and professional caregivers may differ in home and community settings (Paulus, van Raak, & Keijzer, 2005).

We argue that consideration of fit or match between services and needs of the family caregiver and care recipient, mutuality or collaboration in relationships between family caregivers and professionals, and attention to changes in the needs of family caregivers and their relative over time may be more important to service for and research on family caregiving than tracking the specific tasks done by either family or professionals. As Sin (2006) has suggested, the distinction between formal and informal sources of support makes a limited contribution to in-depth understanding the experience of family caregivers.

In conclusion, our research findings on caregivers' experience of support from professionals suggest that, for family caregivers, mutuality is a valued and important component of their interactions with professionals. Caregivers seek support that is a good fit with their perception of the needs of their relative or themselves, but they often experience support resources that do not match their requirements. Although caregivers experience support from both family and friends and professionals, we argue for viewing support of family caregivers from an integrative perspective that avoids classification of sources of support into formal (professional) or informal (family) categories.

NOTE

The data reported in this chapter were drawn from the studies of women and men caregivers that were reported in the following publications: Coe & Neufeld (1999) and Heinrich, Neufeld, & Harrison (2003).

REFERENCES

Badr, H., Acitelli, L., Duck, S., & Carl, W. (2001). Weaving social support and relationships together. In B. Sarason & S. Duck (Eds.), *Personal relationships: Implications for clinical and community psychology* (pp. 1–14). New York: Wiley.

Brown, J. W., Chen, S., Mitchell, C., & Province, A. (2007). Help-seeking by older husbands caring for wives with dementia. *Journal of Advanced Nursing, 59*(4), 352–360.

Carpentier, N., & Ducharme, F. (2003). Caregiver network transformations: The need for an integrated perspective. *Ageing & Society, 23*, 507–525.

Chappell, N., & Blandford, A. (1991). Informal and formal care: Exploring complementarity. *Ageing & Society, 11*(3), 299–317.

Coe, M., & Neufeld, A. (1999). Male caregivers' use of formal support. *Western Journal of Nursing Research, 2*(4), 568–588.

Collins, C., King, S., Given, C. W., & Given, B. (1994). When is a service a service?: Understanding community service use among family caregivers of Alzheimer's patients. In E. Light, G. Niederehe, & B. D. Lebowitz (Eds.), *Stress effects on family caregivers of Alzheimer's patients* (pp. 316–329). New York: Springer.

Cook, K. S., & Emerson, R. M. (1978). Power, equity and commitment in exchange networks. *American Sociological Review, 43*, 721–739.

Cook, K. S., & Rice, E. (2003). Social exchange theory. In J. Delamater (Ed.), *Handbook of social psychology* (pp. 53–76). New York: Kluwer Academic/Plenum.

Dehle, C., Larsen, D., & Landers, J. E. (2001). Social support in marriage. *American Journal of Family Therapy, 29*, 307–324.

Dellasega, C., & Mastrian, K. (1995). The process and consequences of institutionalizing an elder. *Western Journal of Nursing Research, 17*(2), 123–136.

Dupuis, S., & Norris, J. (1997). A multidimensional and contextual framework for understanding diverse family members' roles in long-term care facilities. *Journal of Aging Studies, 11*(4), 297–325.

Eales, J., Keating, N., & Damsma, A. (2001). Seniors' experiences of client-centred residential care. *Ageing & Society, 21*, 279–296.

Edelman, P., & Hughes, S. (1990). The impact of community care on provision of informal care to homebound elderly persons. *Journal of Gerontology: Social Sciences, 45*, S574–S584.

Fisher, E. B. (1997). Two approaches to social support in smoking cessation: Commodity model and nondirective support. *Addictive Behaviors, 22*, 819–833.

Fisher, E. B., LaGreca, A. M., Greco, P., Arfken, C., & Schneiderman, N. (1997). Directive and nondirective support in diabetes management. *International Journal of Behavioral Medicine, 4,* 131–144.

Gladstone, J., & Wexler, E. (2002). Exploring the relationships between families and staff caring for residents in long-term care facilities: Family members' perspectives. *Canadian Journal on Aging, 21*(1), 39–46.

Guberman, N., & Maheu, P. (2002). Conceptions of family caregivers: Implications for professional practice. *Canadian Journal on Aging, 21*(1), 27–37.

Haesler, E., Bauer, M., & Nay, R. (2007). Staff–family relationships in the care of older people: A report on a systematic review. *Research in Nursing & Health, 30,* 385–398.

Harber, K. D., Schneider, J. K., Everard, K. M., & Fisher, E. B. (2005). Directive support, nondirective support, and morale. *Journal of Social and Clinical Psychology, 24,* 691–722.

Hayes, P. (2006). Home is where their health is: Rethinking perspectives of informal and formal care by older rural Appalachian women who live alone. *Qualitative Health Research, 16*(2), 282–297.

Heinrich, M., Neufeld, A., & Harrison, M. J. (2003). Seeking support: Caregivers' strategies for interacting with health personnel. *Canadian Journal of Nursing Research, 35*(4), 39–56.

Hertzberg, A., & Ekman, S. (2000). "We, not them and us?": Views on the relationships and interactions between staff and relatives of older people permanently living in nursing homes. *Journal of Advanced Nursing, 31,* 614–622.

Hurley, A., Volicer, L., Rempusheski, V., & Fry, S. (1995). Reaching consensus: The process of commending treatment decisions for Alzheimer's patients. *Advances in Nursing Science, 18*(2), 33–43.

Kaye, L. W., & Applegate, J. S. (1990). Contributions to care from the outside. In L. Kaye & J. S. Applegate (Eds.), *Men as caregivers to the elderly* (pp. 47–85). Toronto, ON: Lexington Books.

Legault, A. & Ducharme, F. (2009). Advocating for a parent with dementia in a long-term care facility. *Journal of Family Nursing, 15,* 198–219.

Lindgren, C. L. (1993). The caregiver career. *Image: Journal of Nursing Scholarship, 25*(3), 214–219.

Litwak, E. (1985). *Helping the elderly: The complementary roles of informal networks and formal systems.* New York: Guilford.

Lyons, K., & Zarit, S. (1999). Formal and informal support: The great divide. *International Journal of Geriatric Psychiatry, 14,* 183–196.

Molm, L., Peterson, G., & Takahashi, N. (1999). Power in negotiated and reciprocal exchange. *American Sociological Review, 64,* 876–890.

Molm, L. D., Quist, T. M., & Wisely, P. A. (1994). Imbalanced structures, unfair strategies: Power and justice in social exchange. *American Sociological Review, 59,* 98–121.

Paulus, A., van Raak, A., & Keijzer, F. (2005). Informal and formal caregivers' involvement in nursing home activities: Impact of integrated care. *Journal of Advanced Nursing, 49*(4), 354–366.

Penning, M. J. (2002). Hydra revisited: Substituting formal for self- and informal in-home care among older adults with disabilities. *The Gerontologist, 42*(1), 4–16.

Rafaeli, E., & Gleason, M. E. J. (2009). Skilled support within intimate relationships. *Journal of Family Theory & Review, 1,* 20–37.

Robinson, K. M., Buckwalter, K. C., & Reed, D. (2005). Predictors of use of services among dementia caregivers. *Western Journal of Nursing Research, 27*(2), 126–140.

Sebern, M. (2005). Shared care, elder and family member skills to manage burden. *Journal of Advanced Nursing, 52*(2), 170–179.

Sin, C. H. (2006). Expectations of support among White British and Asian-Indian older people in Britain: The interdependence of formal and informal spheres. *Health and Social Care in the Community, 14,* 215–224.

Stommel, M., Collins, C., Given, B. A., & Given, C. W. (1999). Correlates of community service attitudes among family caregivers. *Journal of Applied Gerontology, 18*(2), 145–161.

Walker, E., & Jane Dewar, B. (2001). How do we facilitate carers' involvement in decision making? *Journal of Advanced Nursing, 34,* 329–337.

Ward-Griffin, C., & McKeever, P. (2000). Relationships between nurses and family caregivers: Partners in care? *Advances in Nursing Science, 22*(3), 88–103.

Willoughby, J., & Keating, N. (1991). Being in control: The process of caring for a relative with Alzheimer's disease. *Qualitative Health Research, 1,* 27–50.

Wilson, H. S. (1989). Family caregiving for a relative with Alzheimer's dementia: Coping with negative choices. *Nursing Research, 38,* 94–98.

Winslow, B. W. (2003). Family caregivers' experiences with community services: A qualitative analysis. *Public Health Nursing, 20*(5), 341–348.

Wuest, J., Ericson, P. K., & Stern, P. N. (1994). Becoming strangers: The changing family care-giving relationship in Alzheimer's disease. *Journal of Advanced Nursing, 20,* 437–443.

6

Social Support and Caregiving in the Context of Migration

Immigration and culture are influences that affect the experience of support among family caregivers. Global migration is one of the prominent demographic features of North American society and often requires the reconfiguration or renegotiation of familial and gender roles as immigrants encounter competing values and demands. Our research with immigrant women in Canada was undertaken to examine the context for family caregiving by exploring the intersections of gender, family caregiving, and migration and by examining how immigrant women established connections with sources of social support. In our study, we focused on immigrant women from two of the most prominent source regions for migrants to Canada, Chinese East Asia, and South Asia. In this chapter, we first examine the context of migration as an influence on the experience of support among South Asian immigrant women in Canada while caregiving and then discuss our findings of their caregiving experience and ability to establish linkages with potential sources of support. We well understand that others may wish to use this discussion as a means to understand social support and caregiving in the context of their own local situation. We welcome such reflection but also note the distinctive characteristics that may prevail in any one locale.

FAMILY CAREGIVING IN THE CONTEXT OF MIGRATION

Women's caregiving is central to the practice of culturally appropriate roles that serve to differentiate ethnic boundaries and sustain traditional beliefs against competing values that threaten transnational communities with dissolution. The role of caregiving in shaping individual, gender, and group identity is so essential that these activities can be acknowledged within communities of migrants as exhausting or constraining, but not as burdensome or oppressive. These issues, however, can be weighty for individual women. As a 29-year-old Chinese caregiver who joined her husband's family in Canada, said:

> I really don't know what to do. I really adjust to a big family. Before I was married, I was happy with my husband. After, I felt there are lots of burden on my shoulder. Well, I am kind of person. I try to change myself to adjust to the environment. Also, what can I say? Can I say I want to get divorced? I want to walk away from my husband? I cannot go anywhere. One expression in Chinese, "My wings have been cut; where can I fly?"

On the basis of our ethnographic research with Chinese and South Asian women caring for children or adult relatives with health problems, we argue that family caregiving is problematic for immigrant women who attempt to fulfill cultural expectations in a context of altered resources associated with migration. Often migrant women have fewer kin to rely on and lack access to extra household laborers, who would commonly share domestic responsibilities in their home country. An unanticipated decline in socioeconomic status frequently leads to increased participation of immigrant women in the paid labor force, further compressing the time available to conduct household tasks and to fulfill their duties as caregivers. Cultural values such as filial piety, dharma, familism, and cultural ways of relating to others have been found to remain at the core of immigrant women's caregiving activities (Jones, Zhang, Jaceldo-Siegl, & Meleis, 2002; Team, Markovic, & Manderson, 2007). Consequently, women's role in the transmission of culture often does not allow for any significant renegotiation of these duties; redistribution of caregiving responsibilities may fail to occur, and assistance outside the family may not be utilized.

BACKGROUND: CAREGIVING, GENDER, SOCIAL, AND CULTURAL CONTEXTS

The association of caregiving labor with women's gender roles is widespread, yet cultural and religious values also influence the value and appraisal of family caregiving (Brewer, 2001; George, 1998; Limpanichkul & Magilvy, 2004; Remennick, 1999; Team, Markovic, & Manderson, 2007). For example, the construction of caregiving responsibilities as burdensome differs among cultural groups (Asahara, Momose, Murashima, Okubo, & Magilvy, 2001; Martin, 2000; Tirrito & Nathanson, 1994). In some societies, neglect of caregiving responsibilities, not the burden of the caregiving duties themselves, can elicit negative responses. In Vietnam, Japan, and Taiwan, for example, failure to engage appropriately in family caregiving or even efforts to obtain assistance of formal support services can be regarded as a failure that can bring shame to one's family and community (Asahara et al., 2001; Braun, Takamura, & Mougeot, 1996; Hsu & Shyu, 2003). Although caregiving may be difficult, for many the enactment of the role brings self-satisfaction and the recognition of others (Chao & Roth, 2000; Gelfand & McCallum, 1994; Jones, 1996). Some studies suggest that cultural appraisal of the value of caregiving may mediate the effects of caregiving stress (Aranda & Knight, 1997; Connell & Gibson, 1997; Scharlach et al., 2006) that otherwise contributes to the deterioration of the physical and psychological health of caregivers (Lee, 1999). Notably, gender and ethnicity have been found to be more significant than social class in determining obligations felt toward caring for parents (Stein et al., 1998).

Caring in South Asian society (George, 1998) is embedded in the formation of women's moral and ethical selves. Caring encourages investment in, and loyalty to, the larger kin group. The family can be regarded as the embodiment of a society in which each member fulfills roles to enhance the whole family (Chekki, 1988); familial obligations are therefore expected to supersede personal desires. Although these obligations may be framed within the language of dharma and karma among Hindu South Asians, the sentiments are shared among South Asians of other religious backgrounds (George, 1998).

Among Chinese families, caregiving is an essential element of filial piety that demands service and obedience to ancestors, parents, elders, and officials in exchange for their benevolence and care (Hsü, 1991). Physical, financial, and social sacrifice and the provision of services, the cornerstones of filial piety, are primarily carried out by women, daughters-in-law in particular (Sung, 1991; Youn, Knight, Jeong, & Benton, 1999). The maintenance or accumulation of face, comprised of two elements—*mien-zu,* derived from social acknowledgment, and *lian,* ascribed moral standing—provide the moral persuasion to enact filial obligations (Chang & Holt, 1994; Phillips, 1993). Because of a belief in *yin-guo* (cause and effect), heavy family caregiving may be viewed as repaying the caregiver's debt to the receiver or a way to accumulate blessings, such as a peaceful life (Hsu & Shyu, 2003).

Caregiving responsibilities, however, may assume different import abroad. In multicultural societies, such as Canada, women serve as symbolic markers of ethnicity and are responsible for securing and maintaining the boundaries between their ethnocultural community and "mainstream" Euro-Canadian society (Yuval-Davis, 1997). The gender expectations that define women as family caregivers and require the enactment of filial piety or dharma are maintained through socialization in gender roles and are expressed in terms of kin obligation and duty. Women's internal surveillance mechanisms impel them to fulfill and gain satisfaction from the enactment of caregiving responsibilities. Women are also subject to external surveillance from community members and fear ostracism if they do not enact appropriate roles as dutiful spouse, daughter-in-law, or parent (George, 1998).

THE CANADIAN CONTEXT

Since the 1960s, Canada has embraced multiculturalism, which facilitated the entry of migrants from non-European countries. Moreover, these changes created a policy framework that supports the reunification of families and encourages the entry of skilled labor and entrepreneurs (Simmons, 1999). The policy changes have dramatically altered the demographic and social profile of Canada. In less than 40 years, the source of Canadian immigrants has shifted from Europe to Asia, with China, India, and Pakistan serving as the primary source countries in 1999–2000 (Citizenship and Immigration Canada, 2001).

Economic resources can facilitate women's ability to be caregivers by reducing the need to work outside the home, by enabling the purchase of services, and by providing access to support services available through the employer; however, immigrant women caregivers are generally disadvantaged economically. The Canadian female population of women born outside of Canada is relatively well educated. In 2001, 18% of immigrant women had a university degree, compared with 14% of other women (Statistics Canada, 2006). Nonvisible minority immigrant women catch up to native-born Canadian women in wages after 11 years, but visible minority immigrant women never catch up; overall, the initial discrepancy in the earnings gap between immigrants and Canadian-born workers has widened, and the catch-up to Canadian levels has slowed (Apinunmahakul, Harris, & Meng, 2004). The discrepancy in socioeconomic status between native and foreign-born women is attributable in part to the reluctance of Canadian officials and professionals to recognize foreign credentials and the demand by employers for Canadian job experience. Both of these practices serve to diminish women's ability to procure remunerative work in their field of expertise (Mulvihill, Mailloux, & Atkin, 2001). As a result, immigrant women are concentrated in lower-wage positions in the sales and service industry, although they are often overqualified for these occupations. For instance, university-educated immigrant women are less likely than Canadian-born women to work as professionals or managers and more likely to be found in clerical, sales, and service jobs traditionally held by women (Statistics Canada, 2006).

In the Canadian context, government support is provided for health care and some caregiving activities, the range of which is determined at the provincial level. However, the model of care is still one that depends largely on the care work of immediate female family members (Armstrong & Armstrong, 2001) and is similar to the policy changes in the United Kingdom in recent decades, which support care of older people by family and friends in the community rather than the provision of direct care by government services (Sin, 2006). The policy expectation that women will assume familial caregiving responsibilities can create competing demands for women. The gap in wages between men and women means that women are more likely than their male counterparts to forgo full-time employment to fulfill caregiving responsibilities (Lee, 1999; Luxton & Corman, 2001). However, because many immigrant families face downward mobility and economic strain, relinquishing paid employment is increasingly problematic (Gelfand & McCallum, 1994; Slonim-Nevo, Cwikel, Luski, Lankry, & Shraga, 1995). Furthermore, immigrant women coping with low-waged employment, downward mobility, and caregiving responsibilities, especially those engaged with both child and elder care, have reported increased health problems and stress (Remennick, 1999).

Our research builds on caregiving literature by considering caregiving within the context of the migration process. We examine family caregiving in relation to gender roles and cultural identities, because caregiving can be more intensively charged when these activities are conducted in a migrant community far removed from the country of origin. Ideas about migration have shifted from a focus on uprooting and resettlement, characterized by the severing of homeland ties, to a consideration of migrants as transnationals, part of the flow of people who cross borders in the context of a global economy (Appadurai, 1991), maintain connections with their homelands, and develop complex identities and relations (Basch, Schiller, & Blanc, 1994). The experiences of immigrant family caregivers, therefore, can be understood in the context of the geopolitical forces that have influenced and constrained Asian migration to Canada.

INFLUENCES ON CAREGIVING

Caregiving Beliefs and Women's Roles

In our research, both South Asian and Chinese participants felt that women were the most appropriate caregivers for elders as well as for children. For instance, one 29-year-old Chinese caregiver described how the expectations of her in-laws that she provide extensive care for her father-in-law were based on their view that this was the appropriate role for her as the daughter-in-law.

> They [the husband's family] don't like an outsider to get into the family. They are traditional. They think this is my job and I have to do it.

A university-educated Punjabi woman commented on her obligation as a daughter and daughter-in-law to care for the elders in her family:

> I have two children of my own, and my mother-in-law is living with me. And on the other hand, I have my own parents who are . . . getting old . . . . I'm not responsible directly, but we, I'm an older daughter. . . . I always feel responsible because if anything happens to them emotionally, they call me. So I feel I'm responsible for that too.

Women were regarded as more sensitive than men to the needs of others. A university-educated, middle-class, 37-year-old Chinese woman noted how her 5-year-old daughter recognized the strain caregiving placed on her, vowing to be well behaved so as not to burden her mother any further. Her son did not notice her distress.

> I went back to my parents' house, I found out my, uh, my father's sick again. . . . When I went home, I was not happy. And my daughter noticed. She asked me, "Mom, how come you're not happy?" I was so surprised, only five years old! She knows I'm not happy. I said, "Because, your grandpa is . . . sick . . . so I'm not happy." And she knows. She just told me, "Oh, I'll be good tonight. I won't be fighting with Brother, and, uh, I'll be good to you." But my son, he just, he doesn't even notice.

Despite the expectation that daughters-in-law would care for their elders, the women caring for elders often noted that parents longed for the company of their sons. A Chinese caregiver reflected,

> They only want their son to be with them. Even though he doesn't do much about it.

The majority perspective of our participants was that men were not suited for care work. Because men had predominantly been the recipients of attention and care throughout their lives, they were generally construed as inept in the provision of care. For example, the younger brother of one Chinese caregiver, who is employed full-time, was brought from Hong Kong to help with their parents. He has not, however, found satisfactory work, nor, in her eyes, has he been particularly helpful to the family:

> I be a full-time mom, a full work . . . taking care of my parents. . . . He [a surviving younger brother] is living with my parents. I don't think he can even [be] taking care of himself well enough to [be] taking care of the sick parent.

Both the association of caregiving with women and the construction of men as incompetent in these matters generally prevented both genders from sharing equally in these tasks. Therefore, when a man did offer support to a female relative, it was usually on a limited basis.

Maintaining Cultural Identity

The findings of our research suggest that women, as mothers, are increasingly entrusted with the task of maintaining cultural identity, through educating the young and modeling desired behavior. According to participants in our research, modeling these virtues for their children and others was vital, not only for their own standing within their community but also to engage their children in the network of reciprocity that underscored these values. From the perspective of a 48-year-old recent Chinese immigrant, who is caring for her infirm mother with some support from her brother, the rest of her siblings are disregarding their familial obligations. She explained why she has assumed responsibility for her parent:

> What makes me feel satisfied is that I know how to care for her through filial piety. When I tell the children to treat the elderly nicely, they may say, "What about you?" So there is comparison. I think the most important thing is to accommodate to each other. Sometimes, she takes care of me. Sometimes she waits for an hour. So, this is family love.

A 45-year-old, university-educated, middle-class South Asian woman, caring for her mother and father, also copes with the demands of paid employment, her children and spouse, and housework duties. She reinforced these sentiments:

> I also think the children will learn from my experience that they should respect and help elders.

Most women rejected the idea of caregiving as a burden, despite reporting exhaustion, ill health, and anxiety resulting from the overwhelming duties they must complete. Instead, they perceived caregiving as part of their role within the family and community. The descriptions of two South Asian caregivers and a Chinese caregiver follow.

> Maybe in our culture, and maybe that's why I am looking after my elderly instead of just throwing them into a nursing home. . . . I had to sell my house to move in with them when they became very old, and I didn't really like doing it. But they need the emotional support as well as the physical support. Maybe in our culture people are more sensitive to the elderly. They are not considered garbage. (**South Asian caregiver**)

> Well, it's a member of family, and I take it for granted that he is more comfortable when I can get, when I can give him the care he needs. And in our

family relations, really, we take it for granted that we care for each other. (**South Asian caregiver**)

Filial piety and caring are what we should do. (**Chinese caregiver**)

Even in cases where the care recipient was unpleasant or hostile, some participants felt satisfied that they had fulfilled their obligations in a gracious and appropriate manner. This dedication was contrasted with Euro-Canadian approaches, which, in the view of the immigrant women, seemed to invite greater institutional intervention. When one university-educated, middle-class Chinese caregiver, age 49, was offered the option of institutionalizing her in-laws, she responded,

Lady, you don't know what you're talking about. You come from a different culture where [sic] I came from.

Nevertheless, some women did experience negative outcomes of caregiving. At age 29, a Chinese caregiver described feeling isolated and depressed. A mother of three children, she assists her mother-in-law in caring for her cold and demanding father-in-law.

I am not as happy and free as before. My whole life is around this family.

I don't have friends. I feel I am getting older staying at home all day. I look at myself, I feel so old. . . . I feel like falling from the heaven to the hell.

Immigration, Familial Responsibilities, and Employment

The impact of immigration on women's ability to cope with caregiving responsibilities is significant. Migration often means that familial networks become smaller or dispersed, reducing the numbers of kin that can be called on for support. A 72-year-old South Asian woman compared her experience as a caregiver in India and Canada:

I was looking after my father in India. It seemed that we had more time there. I used to spend lots of time with him, in his last few days. Even my employer gave me lots of free time to spend with him. My uncle stayed with my father for one and a half month; he was in Canada. All the family came, and we stayed together for few weeks. I don't think you can do it here. In India, there is more closeness.

Sponsoring relatives from overseas to care for infirm family members in Canada is not uncommon, but it requires an investment of time and financial resources, because family members who act as immigration sponsors must demonstrate the ability to support incoming relations for several years (Citizenship and Immigration Canada, 2009). These efforts may be too costly for low-income households and too time-consuming for those who require immediate assistance.

South Asian and Chinese Canadian caregivers found themselves balancing the demands of caregiving with the needs of other family members. Although, for some, spousal relations suffered, others said that the presence of a helpful spouse helped ameliorate their distress. A 40-year-old, middle-class Punjabi woman told us,

> I give her [the mother-in-law] bath in the evening. . . . Usually my husband helps out. We have no help from friends or any other family member. I come home in the evening, then prepare supper for the whole family, give bath to my small kids, clean the house.

South Asian and Chinese caregivers found that the presence of kin and their competing demands contributed to stress in Canada, whereas similar interactions in their home countries would have been more supportive or less problematic.

The costs of securing paid assistance with family caregiving tasks are higher in Canada (Bian, 1994; Cheng, 1996). Economic conditions and the Canadian context made it difficult to procure extrafamilial domestic assistance.

> My father was on a very good job back home [India], was in police. We had lots of servants. They did everything. Over here, I have to do everything like cook, clean, work outside the home, look after my children. (**South Asian woman caring for her parents**)

> Labor back where I came from is a lot cheaper. I think I would be able to employ someone full-time . . . even if I were, uh, to apply someone to come . . . from overseas, say, for example, a Filipino maid or something. . . . The regulations are not as tough. It would be faster, it would be easier to get one, and cheaper of course. (**Chinese woman caring for her parents**)

Many women worked outside the home in low-paying jobs to supplement the family income. Their employment status further exacerbated their experience of time compression and demanded well-organized plans to cope with the needs of care recipients and other family members. The woman previously quoted clearly outlined how her day was organized to combine family caregiving and employment outside the home.

> Okay, I get up at 5:00 a.m. Five, every morning, so I have my parents' meal cooked, both breakfast and lunch. I leave the house at 6:30 a.m. for work. I don't come home until 4:00 p.m. Take a shower. That's my best time of the day, myself, I can relax. Maybe a drink of tea. Then I start cooking supper. My supper is at around 7:30 p.m. You know, after wash up everything. Make sure my mom take her pills. Do her night care. Get her up to her room. Make sure she takes all her medication then tuck her into bed, and pray she, that she will sleep the whole night.

Because this caregiver's employment did not offer supplemental health insurance, family benefits, or flexible hours, it was difficult for her to take time off to accompany her parents to appointments or to provide personal care. Other women, such as the 45-year-old South Asian daughter who is quoted as follows, also had little time to pursue avenues of treatment or support for their family member because of their need to work outside the home.

> I had to make time from my work, housework, and kids to take them [the parents] for the fitting of belt and also to check different shops for the walkers to compare their costs.

In summary, the lack of kin support and the demands of often inflexible and poorly waged employment created additional stress for immigrant women caring for family members by increasing demands on their time and financial strain.

Extrafamilial Assistance

With the belief that care is best carried out in the home by family members and limited traditions of accessing services, many of the women chose not to use available formal services. For example, one caregiver works and cares for two children, her father, and her mother, who has diabetes and Alzheimer's disease. Although she feels guilty about attending to the needs of her parents before those of her children, she cannot come to avail herself of services that are culturally and linguistically unacceptable to her parents.

> I always tell myself, this is my own parents. You look after them. No one are [sic] going to help you.

Similarly, a South Asian woman says,

> Care is not . . . to be bought, not a service to be bought. It's a service we have to provide out of our mouth, and affection for the other human being.

Access to the informal support of friends is also inhibited by an in-group orientation that often confined discussion of care recipients' conditions or caregiving stress to household members. For instance, a Chinese caregiver noted that elder family members found inquiries and unsolicited advice from acquaintances to be intrusive.

> My mother-in-law doesn't like people to ask about her grandson's problem. She doesn't like it.

Sharing this information with friends and other community members was seen as creating an unnecessary burden for others, who would be incapable of understanding their situation.

Interviews with participants who cared for children with chronic conditions revealed that immigrant caregivers were more forthcoming in seeking out and using services for their children. Women availed themselves of a variety of services, including special education, hospital-based therapy programs, aids for daily living, and home care services for children. Some women became health advocates, alongside other parents, and actively campaigned for access to specialized services for children in need. One Chinese mother, a 43-year-old university-educated woman, remarked that one formal advocacy group she approached taught her to make demands.

> So it was very hard to, to fight, but the teacher help me to . . . how to appeal and fight . . . for the speech [therapy].

Although the limited number of cases and types of conditions in our research do not allow us to speculate, a mother's ability to consider and effect health care decisions pertaining to her children may be an avenue for migrant women to renegotiate caregiving responsibilities with persons or services external to the family. Moreover, the decision making regarding children may be less burdened by concerns such as an elder's response to outsiders or the cultural appropriateness of health care.

We next discuss how immigrant women sought to establish connections with community sources of support outside the family. Although their cultural preference was to provide family care to family members, the women did need to access services for health care, medical aids, and social programs for their family member. Some of the women also used services that enabled them to continue to care for their family member in their home. Their connections within their social networks, especially ties with others in their ethnic community, were a key bridge in their ability to link with services.

MISSING LINKS AND ESTABLISHING CONNECTIONS WITH COMMUNITY RESOURCES

Almost half the women in our sample did not establish connections with community resources. Those who did, however, established connections with services in their community through their informal social networks, which included relatives, friends, community or church associates, and professionals. We begin this section by discussing the experience of the women in our study who did not report making any connections to community resources.

Absence of Network Ties to Community Resources

Caregivers who were not connected to community resources were particularly vulnerable to lack of support and the associated negative impact on their health. Women in this group included caregivers of an adult or child; recent, intermediate, and long-term immigrants; those who were employed or not employed outside the home; and women whose relatives resided either in the local community or abroad. Of the women who reported no linkage with outside resources, most were interviewed in the language of their country of origin. No identifiable pattern in their access to support was associated with variations in time since immigration, employment, age of care recipient, or geographical location of relatives, nor was there any consistent difference identified between their caregiving situations and the circumstances of women who connected with community resources.

These women provided an example of the isolation of women caregivers. In focus groups with women and professionals, at the end of the study, we invited participants to respond to several composite scenarios. Participants in all of the focus group discussions of scenarios noted the isolation of women caregivers.

> So, it's not only the language, I think she's [the caregiver in a scenario] isolating herself from everybody else . . . she's only connected to her family . . . I don't think she has friends, you know. . . . Because friends will tell you, sometimes . . . or neighbors will. (**Professional service provider in focus group**)

Focus group participants suggested that women may feel trapped, lack connections to others, lack the confidence to make their needs known, or fear disclosure to relatives who might consider them incompetent. Both caregivers and professionals said that, although caregivers needed to take the initiative to seek out resources, community agencies must also adopt initiatives to reach out and connect with immigrant women caregivers. In response to a scenario about a developmentally delayed child, one professional service provider commented in a focus group:

> The key question that we have is . . . how . . . [do] programmers reach the parents?

Relatives, Friends, and Other Caregivers Facilitating Connections

Most women in our study had relatives in the same city, other parts of Canada, and their country of origin, but several made no reference to family members outside of North America. The range of services that they accessed through different patterns of making connections included speech therapy, respite care for an elder, a school for special needs children, or home care for an elder or child.

The most common way for the women to connect with community resources was through relatives and friends in their informal social network. They reported assistance from a friend within their ethnic community who was a social worker, nurse, or physician. Friends with professional backgrounds were able to ensure privacy and interpret expectations and characteristics of community resources in a meaningful way. One caregiver noted that many women who do not have friends in these professional roles do not know what resources are available:

> We have friends who are social workers and who are nurses, who are doctors . . . so, we get to know more about the system, but if you don't know these people . . . sometimes it is really hard to get information. (**Chinese caregiver**)

Connections also occurred when the caregiver knew other family members or caregivers who required similar services. For example, one Chinese caregiver sought assistance for her child from a local rehabilitation center because her niece/nephew also had a developmental delay and had received services there. When asked how she knew of these community services, she responded,

> I didn't know anything. It is only because his other cousin went [to an agency] for the assessment.

Another woman, who was caring for a husband with cancer, appreciated a church member's recommendation that she contact a Chinese medical practitioner. She was frustrated with her husband's inability to eat and the difficult challenge of cooking meals he could tolerate.

> He couldn't eat again. He couldn't take the nutrients. . . . He [was] referred by a friend in the Church. . . . We cannot just take the prescription and get the herbal medicine here. If the person in the Church doesn't know the doctor, we won't be able to know this doctor [a Chinese medical practitioner]. (**Chinese caregiver**)

One mother reported asking other caregivers in her ethnic community for information when she needed a wheelchair for her son. These inquiries helped her recognize the advantages and disadvantages of different alternatives. In her case, this support from other family caregivers supplemented the information and advice that was available to her from a social worker.

A Chain of Linkages to Community Resources

Some women described a chain of linkages between friends, relatives, other caregivers, health and social service professionals, and community resources. The process involved one contact, sometimes unrelated to caregiving, leading to another contact and, ultimately, to access to community resources. For example, a mother described how first a friend in a parenting class and then her child's teacher commented on her child's slow development. Through the teacher's recommendation that she contact her family physician, the mother was eventually connected with appropriate services.

> They have parenting class, and I attend that and I get some friend, and then get some teachers. They [teacher] told me he seems to have some problem. They suggest me talk to the family doctor and then the family doctor command me to go to the [rehabilitation center]. (**Chinese caregiver**)

In another situation, the aunt of a woman caregiver referred her to respite services for her elderly mother; the respite service, in turn, became a link to other community resources. When asked how she discovered these community services, the caregiver replied,

> From the respite home. And this information, actually about the respite home, the aunt mentioned to me. That's how we came to know other departments. And then you come to know more and more. (**South Asian caregiver**)

Contact with one community resource provided a bridge to other resources—through referral, advocacy support, and distribution of information. For example, one mother with assistance from an advocacy association for handicapped children successfully appealed the denial of her application for financial assistance from a government program:

> So I talk to them [association for handicapped children] . . . and then they just said you know, if you need it you have to fight because they don't give you that easy . . . they help me to do with the appeal. (**Chinese caregiver**)

Influence of Cultural Beliefs in Negotiating Access to Resources

Immigrant women's beliefs sometimes restricted access to support from community resources. For example, women who valued privacy were reluctant to disclose personal problems and feelings to a stranger. One caregiver observed that a more indirect form of communication with a friend within her ethnic community, who was also a professional, overcame both the language barrier and concerns about privacy while gaining her access to expert information. For another family, reluctance to disclose the nature of a child's developmental delay, because of a concern that this would reflect negatively on the family, precluded a request for assistance. The child's grandmother believed that no one outside the family should care for her developmentally delayed grandson.

> Sometimes we also ask our relatives to take care of our son. If we cannot find any family member we would pay school teachers . . . my mother-in-law worries if an outsider takes care of the son. (**Chinese caregiver**)

A South Asian woman in the focus group discussion also noted that a child with a developmental delay would stigmatize the whole family.

These women's strong commitment to their responsibility to care for their relative, often described as filial piety by the Chinese women, also influenced their access to community resources. One Chinese caregiver described her frustration that no home care assistance could be obtained for her parents, who lived with her; they would be eligible only if they lived alone. This policy conflicted with her commitment to care for them:

> They're living with me. If I dumped them out, leave them outside on their own, I'm sure they will get some help. But this is my parents I am talking about. You think I can do that to them?

Conflict between beliefs in traditional herbal medicine and Western medicine created a dilemma for some Chinese women. The parents-in-law of a Chinese woman were the primary caregivers of her developmentally delayed son for 5 years while she and her husband worked abroad. When she returned, she wanted to consult a traditional Chinese medical practitioner for her son, but her mother-in-law objected on the grounds that the child might have a reaction to any herbs prescribed. Although the mother considered treating the child secretly, she decided that this would reflect disrespect for her parents-in-law.

> Although he is my son, he is also like my in-laws' son. Sometimes my friends referred Chinese medicine to me . . . my mother-in-law would say "Don't give this poor kid any medication". . . . At first I plan to take my son to see this doctor secretly . . . my friends also referred acupuncture to me. I took my son there around one year. (**Chinese caregiver**)

A Chinese caregiver agonized over her lack of knowledge of Western medicine. Her grandmother had a fall and was treated by a traditional Chinese herbalist for a year without improvement. She later discovered that her grandmother had had a fracture, and it was no longer possible to correct her immobility:

> She could not get up after she fell. Maybe we did not know the bone was broken. We brought her to see the herbalist for one year. At the end she could not walk. I did not know until I work here [nursing unit] that we should not move the old people when they fell.

Previous experience in their country of origin can also affect caregivers' perspectives on community resources. One woman noted that, because they were pleased to receive—at no cost—health care services that would not be available in Hong Kong, they did not seek other services. This was reinforced by a professional, who noted in a focus group that families that had been very self-reliant in their home country might not consider seeking help from community services.

Women were also hampered in their ability to access services by inadequate skill in English, even when they had attempted to learn the language. Previously, only one member of a couple, usually the husband, was granted status under the Canadian independent immigration category that provided access to language support (Boyd, 1997; Ng, 1993). This practice occurred even when both husband and wife had comparable education and work experience. More recently, free language instruction has been made available through Citizenship and Immigration Canada to all adult family members (Citizenship and Immigration Canada, 2004, 2007). Despite the increased availability of language education, short programs offered to newcomers can be inadequate for acquiring the level of language that is necessary.

When I first came here I went there to learn English for like several weeks, but now I forgot most of it. (**Chinese caregiver**)

One woman was unable to apply for a walking aid because she could not communicate either her health care number or her name over the phone to the intake worker. Although our primary focus was on initial access to community resources, there is substantial evidence in the data that facility in English is also important in sustaining a beneficial connection with a community service.

If he stays in the hospital or senior center, he needs somebody to speak Mandarin or Taiwanese. If the agent [agency] doesn't provide such service, he prefers staying in the house. (**Chinese caregiver**)

In another situation, the family member who acted as an interpreter lacked the complex English vocabulary necessary to understand the medical terminology used by the specialist. Consequently, the caregiver and family were unable to understand their relative's condition and avoid preventable complications of diabetes. Inadequate skill in English was also a barrier to expressing emotion. As one woman said, "It's hard to use English to talk about emotional needs."

Women also noted that the inability to speak English could limit their choice of potential professionals, such as social workers. Both women and professionals in group discussions referred to the difficulty in assessing children's speech and language development accurately when two languages are involved.

These findings provide insight into the social and cultural context of family members caring for Chinese and South Asian immigrant women. For immigrant women, social networks were important in establishing access to support from community resources but were influenced by migration and women's material circumstances.

DISCUSSION

The experiences of South Asian and Chinese immigrant women caregivers in Canada revealed similar responses, despite differences in culture and the length of residency in Canada. Kin work remains central to women's roles in maintaining cultural identity and familial survival in a transnational community. We found that women were regarded

as natural and appropriate family caregivers who experienced significant strain juggling the competing demands of work and multiple generations of family in a new environment (Gelfand & McCallum, 1994;
Remennick, 1999; Slonim-Nevo et al., 1995). Despite these considerable pressures, the women we interviewed rejected the notion of a caregiving burden, focusing instead on the rewarding aspects of caregiving
obtained through cultural role fulfillment (Chao & Roth, 2000; Gelfand
& McCallum, 1994; Jones, 1996). In the interest of maintaining cultural
values and identity, women did not want, nor were they able, to renegotiate their caregiving roles.

Caregiving, a central focus of kin work, is embedded in a woman's
gender role as wife, mother, and moral being; caregiving responsibilities reinforce gender roles and propagate the values of filial piety and
dharma in Chinese and South Asian families. In transnational communities, the demand to maintain cultural boundaries and values of home
and community on foreign soil depends on the performance of culturally appropriate gender roles whose enactment is both internalized and
scrutinized by others in the community at home and abroad (Alicea,
1997). Interactions with elder generations further ensures adherence to
appropriate behavior. The significance of women's caregiving work to
cultural and gender identity is reflected in the fact that our participants
echoed these sentiments regardless of length of residency in Canada.
Our finding is supported by research in the United States with Chinese
elders in Boston (Aroian, Wu, & Tran, 2005) and by a review of research
on the impact of race, culture, and/or ethnicity on dementia caregiving
that found that non-white caregivers, in comparison to white caregivers,
expressed stronger beliefs about filial support and that, in comparison to
black caregivers, Hispanic caregivers endorsed stronger views on filial
support (Connell & Gibson, 1997).

Other studies have found that there is a gradual change in preference
for care provided by family that correlates with longer residence in the
country of immigration. In a study of Korean immigrants in the United
States (Han, Choi, Kim, Lee, & Kim, 2008), family caregivers described
a preference for adult children to live with and care for their elderly
parents, but individuals who had been in the country for many years also
reported concern that this arrangement might not be feasible if elderly
parents are left alone, because the younger generation need to work
outside the home. Sin (2006) reported a preference among Asian Indian
men and women in the United Kingdom for care provided by family for
older people, but these respondents also commented that government-

funded services may be needed if their children were unable to provide the support. In another study, Asian American women, most of whom were immigrants, described a continuous adjustment of values, as they tried to live by two sets of standards: one reflecting their country of origin and the other reflecting American culture (Jones et al., 2002). The authors in the latter study described the women as moderately acculturated, and the length of residence in the United States ranged from 2 to 46 years.

The expectations of the Chinese and South Asian communities that women should provide care for elders or children are congruent with the perspective of exchange theory, because it is expected that the assistance mothers give their children early in life will be reciprocated by their daughters-in-law (or daughters) in later life (Blau, 1986; Homans, 1961). An indication that women were mindful of this expectation is reflected in the comment of one Chinese woman in our study, who found satisfaction in being a model for her children through her caregiving. She valued the gestures of care that her infirm mother expressed toward her in return as reciprocal and as a part of family love. For Chinese and South Asian women, these expectations were embedded in the cultural and moral values of their heritage and reinforced through a history of relationships between generations.

An interview study of exchange and reciprocity among elderly Japanese and American women identified differences in perceptions (Akiyama, Antonucci, & Campbell, 1997). In response to hypothetical exchanges between older women and their daughters or daughters-in-law, researchers found acceptance of a higher level of dependence by Japanese women in comparison to American women. American women emphasized more symmetry in reciprocity that suppressed one-way transactions, thus reducing dependency and viewing inability to maintain reciprocity as disruptive to the relationship.

Although our study included only women immigrants from China and South Asia, the importance of giving back to family members who had previously provided care and support is a value that is also held by Asian men. Immigrant Korean men who were caring for their ailing spouses in the United States valued the support of their spouses in the past and were able to find positive meaning in their caregiving (Han et al., 2008).

The preference for care provided by family with related values on giving back to others, especially parents who provided care in the past, is shared by others, including Hispanic and African Americans

(Scharlach et al., 2006) and may be associated with religious values for caring (Limpanichkul & Magilvy, 2004; Team, Markovic, & Manderson, 2007). Variations in the social networks of caregivers of elders from different racial and ethnic minorities, and differences in comparison to the networks of white caregivers, also were found in a review of research on family caregiving (Dilworth-Anderson, Williams, & Gibson, 2002). Although the review did not address immigration, it did provide evidence of the influence of cultural values and norms on caregiving, including beliefs about reciprocity, filial obligation, and a sense of responsibility to care for older family members.

When immigrant women caregivers in our research required assistance from outside the family, social ties were a link to community resources. However, some women remained isolated and disconnected. Because they usually entered Canada through the family reunification program, immigrant women caregivers' social networks comprised a few close ties with relatives who had immigrated at an earlier time and assisted them during the early settlement period. They lacked diverse social networks that included connections with others holding divergent views. Although informal support networks can be a screening and referral agent for community resources, there are suggestions that small, high-density networks of strong ties with similar others can act as a barrier to outside help (Grant & Wenger, 1993).

Homogeneous social networks can be barriers, because those with strong ties, such as a common ethnic heritage, often share an overlapping circle of friends and have limited exposure to new information. Conversely, heterogeneous networks of weak ties among acquaintances provide important bridges to wider sources of advice and help than what is available from members of homogeneous networks (Granovetter, 1973). The influence of the social network derives from the beliefs communicated by influential others and from the strength of the tie (Pescosolido, 1991, 1992). In a study of migration in Taiwan, Pescosolido (1986) found that, as contact with others outside the ethnic community increased, migrants eventually adopted views similar to those held by others in their community. For example, those in urban areas accepted Western medicine, whereas migrants to rural areas retained a commitment to traditional practices.

In the absence of strong connections with people outside their ethnic communities, caregivers in this study, as in other research, lacked essential information (Lynam, 1985; Merrell, Kinsella, Murphy, Philpin, & Ali, 2005). The absence of diverse social networks for women may have contributed in part to the dissonance they experienced between their personal values and mainstream professional values with respect to desirable community supports. Dissonance, which has also been identified by others (Anderson, 1991; Lalond, Taylor, & Moghaddam, 1992; Meleis, 1991; Tabora & Flaskerud, 1997), was particularly evident for women caring for elders and restricted their access to community resources. To establish diverse social networks of weak ties, opportunities to form such linkages must be available. In our research, women caregivers described expanding their knowledge through contact with health care agencies, language training, professional education programs, and parenting classes. In addition, ties with friends from their ethnic community who were health or social service professionals provided women with broader access to information about mainstream health and social service resources in the absence of access to a diverse social network. These findings confirm those of others, who have found that family caregivers who have contact with a supportive general practitioner (Merrell et al., 2005) and that those with the opportunity to form weak ties and a more diverse network had a gateway to other connections (Rose, Carrasco, & Charboneau, 1998) and information about community services.

There may be other reasons for the lack of contact with community services. Immigrant women, whose culture and country of origin view caregiving as a natural role for women in families, may not seek out information on community services because they share the belief that caregiving is their family role and responsibility. Team, Markovic, and Manderson (2007) found that Russian-speaking immigrant women in Australia did not attempt to access financial aid for which they were eligible, but they accepted a gendered and private nature for family caregiving, based on the social policies of their countries of origin. Others (Lawrence, Murray, Samsi, & Banerjee, 2008) found that men and women caregivers in the United Kingdom who held what they labeled as traditional caregiver ideology—that is, viewed being a caregiver as natural and virtuous—were likely to put limits on support from health and social agencies. In their study, the majority of South Asian caregivers, in comparison to half of the black Caribbean and a minority of white British caregivers, possessed a traditional ideology. In a study conducted in South Wales, the majority of Bangladeshi informal caregivers held the view that help outside the family for personal care for their adult relative was not acceptable, and consequently they did not seek assistance (Merrell et al., 2005).

We raise a caution in relation to our findings. Our focus was on the experience of immigrant women, but we should be cautious in interpreting their experience exclusively in terms of the experience of migration or cultural values. Although exacerbated by issues of immigration and inadequate language skills, the experience of immigrant women in this study is similar to that of Canadian-born caregivers (Harrison & Neufeld, 1997), particularly those who have low incomes, jobs with limited flexibility, and heavy caregiving demands (Gignac, Kelloway, & Gottlieb, 1996; Gottlieb, Kelloway, & Fraboni, 1994). This study included immigrant women from two of the most dominant immigrant groups in our local area but omitted other immigrant groups, including those who are English speaking and would not experience the same challenges with language, although they may have similar experience in the dispersion and loss of family networks. There is a risk of stereotypically explaining the experience of immigrant women—based on culture, immigration, or lack of facility in the language—without considering the influence of other conditions, such as poverty or loss of family networks. Nevertheless, it is important that health and social services practitioners recognize that a match between the cultural values of family caregivers and the approach of community services is needed to ensure that immigrant caregivers can obtain support that they will use. When caregivers hold the view that their role is to provide family care, they may not be willing to ask for support for themselves, but they may be willing to accept assistance if the service is viewed as helping them provide the care they wish to give.

In conclusion, our research with immigrant women caregivers illustrates the influence of their beliefs and expectations as well as the material, socioeconomic conditions and disruptions that they encountered in the process of migration on their experience of support while caring for a relative. Their social networks and their beliefs about culture and caregiving were pivotal in their access to resources, but immigrant women often struggled alone without resources to fulfill their family commitments. Although findings from other research with ethnically diverse caregiving populations (e.g., Sharlach et al., 2006) are congruent with our research, it is also important to consider, in addition to caregivers' beliefs, the impact of conditions such as poverty or family disruption that are often associated with immigration.

NOTE

The data reported in this chapter were drawn from a study of immigrant women caregivers that was reported in the following publications: Neufeld, Harrison, Stewart, Hughes, & Spitzer (2002) and Spitzer, Neufeld, Harrison, Hughes, & Stewart (2003).

REFERENCES

Akiyama, H., Antonucci, T., & Campbell, R. (1997). Exchange and reciprocity among two generations of Japanese and American women. In J. Sokolovsky (Ed.) *The cultural context of aging: World perspectives* (2nd ed., pp. 163–178). Westport, CT: Greenwood Press.

Alicea, M. (1997). "A chambered nautilus": The contradictory nature of Puerto Rican women's roles in the social construction of a transnational community. *Gender & Society, 11*, 597–626.

Anderson, J. M. (1991). Immigrant women speak of chronic illness: The social construction of the devalued self. *Journal of Advanced Nursing, 16*(6), 710–717.

Appadurai, A. (1991). Global ethnoscapes: Notes and queries for a transnational anthropology. In R. Fox. (Ed.), *Recapturing anthropology: Working in the present* (pp. 191–210). Santa Fe, NM: School of American Research Press.

Apinunmahakul, A., Harris, E., & Meng, P. (2004). *The contribution of social capital to the wages of immigrant and native born Canadians.* Unpublished manuscript, University of Windsor at Windsor, Ontario. Retrieved June 11, 2009 from http://international.metropolis.net

Aranda, M. P., & Knight, B. G. (1997). The influence of ethnicity and culture on the caregiver stress and coping process: A sociocultural review and analysis. *The Gerontologist, 37*(3), 342–354.

Aroian, K. J., Wu, B., & Tran, T. V. (2005). Health care and social service use among Chinese immigrant elders. *Research in Nursing & Health, 28*, 95–105.

Armstrong, P., & Armstrong, H. (2001). *Thinking it through: Women, work and caring in the new millennium.* Halifax, Canada: Maritime Centre of Excellence for Women's Health.

Asahara, K., Momose, Y., Murashima, S., Okubo, N., & Magilvy, J. (2001). The relationship of social norms to use of services and caregiver burden in Japan. *Journal of Nursing Scholarship, 4*, 375–380.

Basch, L., Schiller, N. G., & Blanc, N. S. (1994). *Nations unbound: Transnational projects, postcolonial predicaments and de-territorialized nation-states.* Langhorne, PA: Gordon and Breach.

Bian, Y. (1994). *Work and inequality in urban China.* Albany: State University of New York Press.

Blau, P. M. (1986). *Exchange and power in social life.* New Brunswick, NJ: Transaction Books.

Boyd, M. (1997). Migration policy, female dependency and family membership: Canada and Germany. In P. Evans & G. Wekerle (Eds.), *Women and the Canadian welfare state: Challenges and changes* (pp. 142–169). Toronto, Canada: University of Toronto Press.

Braun, K., Takamura, J., & Mougeot, T. (1996). Perceptions of dementia, caregiving, and help-seeking among recent Vietnamese immigrants. *Journal of Cross-Cultural Gerontology, 11*, 213–228.

Brewer, L. (2001). Gender socialization and the cultural construction of elder caregivers. *Journal of Aging Studies, 15*(3), 217–236.

Chang, H., & Holt, G. R. (1994). A Chinese perspective on face as inter-relational. In S. Ting-Toomey (Ed.), *The challenge of facework: Cross-cultural and interpersonal issues* (pp. 95–132). Albany: State University of New York Press.

Chao, S. Y., & Roth, P. (2000). The experiences of Taiwanese women caring for parents-in-law. *Journal of Advanced Nursing, 31*(3), 631–638.

Chekki, D. (1988). Family in India and North America: Change and continuity among the Lingayat families. *Journal of Comparative Family Studies, 19*(2), 329–343.

Cheng, S. A. (1996). Migrant women domestic workers in Hong Kong, Singapore and Taiwan: A comparative analysis. *Asian and Pacific Migration Journal, 5*(1), 139–152.

Citizenship & Immigration Canada. (2001). *Pursuing Canada's commitment to immigration: The immigration plan for 2002.* Ottawa: Minister of Public Works and Government Services Canada.

———. (2004). *Evaluation of the language instruction for newcomers to Canada (LINC) program.* Retrieved June 11, 2009 from http://www.cic.gc.ca/english/resources/evaluation/linc

———. (2007). *Welcome to Canada: What you should know.* Retrieved June 11, 2009 from http://www.cic.gc.ca/english/resources/publications/welcome

———. (2009). *Sponsoring your family.* Ottawa: Minister of Citizenship, Immigration and Multiculturalism: Canada. Retrieved June 11, 2009 from http://www.cic.gc.ca/english/immigrate/sponsor

Connell, C. M., & Gibson, G. D. (1997). Racial, ethnic and cultural differences in dementia caregiving: Review and analysis. *The Gerontologist, 37*(3), 355–364.

Dilworth-Anderson, P., Williams, I. C., & Gibson, B. (2002). Issues of race, ethnicity, and culture in caregiving research: A 20-year review (1980–2000). *The Gerontologist, 42*(2), 237–272.

Gelfand, D. E., & McCallum, J. (1994). Immigration, the family and female caregivers in Australia. *Journal of Gerontological Social Work, 22*(3/4), 41–59.

George, U. (1998). Caring and women of colour: Living the intersecting oppressions of race, class and gender. In T. Baines, P. M. Evans, & S. Neysmith (Eds.), *Women's caring: Feminist perspectives on social welfare* (pp. 69–83). Oxford, UK: Oxford University Press.

Gignac, M., Kelloway, K., & Gottlieb, B. (1996). The impact of caregiving on employment: A mediational model of work-family conflict. *Canadian Journal on Aging, 15*(4), 525–542.

Gottlieb, B., Kelloway, K., & Fraboni, M. (1994). Aspects of eldercare that place employees at risk. *The Gerontologist, 34*(6), 815–821.

Granovetter, M. S. (1973). The strength of weak ties. *American Journal of Sociology, 78*(6), 1360–1380.

Grant, G., & Wenger, C. (1993). Dynamics of support networks: Differences and similarities between vulnerable groups. *Irish Journal of Psychology, 14*(1), 79–98.

Han, H.-R. Choi, Y. J., Kim, M. T., Lee, J. E., & Kim, K. B. (2008). Experiences and challenges of informal caregiving for Korean immigrants. *Journal of Advanced Nursing, 63,* 517–526.

Harrison, M. J., & Neufeld, A. (1997). Women's experiences of barriers to support while caregiving. *Health Care for Women International, 18*(6), 591–602.

Hsu, H.-C. & Shyu, Y.-I. L. (2003). Implicit exchanges in family caregiving for frail elders in Taiwan. *Qualitative Health Research, 13,* 1078–1093.

Hsü, J. C. H. (1991). Unwanted children and parents: Archaeology, epigraphy and the myths of filial piety. In J. Ching & R. W. L. Guisso (Eds.), *Sages and filial sons: Mythol-*

ogy and archaeology in ancient China (pp. 23–42). Hong Kong: Chinese University of Hong Kong.

Homans, G. C. (1961). *Social behaviour and its elementary forms.* New York: Harcourt, Brace and World.

Jones, P. S. (1996). Asian American women caring for elderly parents. *Journal of Family Nursing, 2*(1), 56–75.

Jones, P. S., Zhang, W. E., Jaceldo-Siegl, & Meleis, A. I. (2002). Caregiving between two cultures: An integrative experience. *Journal of Transcultural Nursing, 13,* 202–209.

Lalond, R. N., Taylor, D. M., & Moghaddam, F. M. (1992). The process of social identification for visible immigrant women in multicultural context. *Journal of Cross-Cultural Psychology, 32*(1), 25–39.

Lawrence, V., Murray, J., Samsi, K., & Banerjee, S. (2008). Attitudes and support needs of Black Caribbean, South Asian and White British carers of people with dementia in the UK. *The British Journal of Psychiatry, 193,* 240–246.

Lee, C. (1999). Health, stress and coping among women caregivers: A review. *Journal of Health Psychology, 4*(1), 27–40.

Limpanichkul, Y., & Magilvy, K. (2004). Managing caregiving at home: Thai caregivers living in the United States, *Journal of Cultural Diversity, 11,* 18–24,

Luxton, M., & Corman, J. (2001). *Getting by in hard times: Gendered labor at home and on the job.* Toronto, Canada: University of Toronto Press.

Lynam, M. J. (1985). Support networks developed by immigrant women. *Social Science & Medicine, 21*(3), 327–333.

Martin, C. D. (2000). More than the work: Race and gender differences in caregiving burden. *Journal of Family Issues, 21*(8), 986–1005.

Meleis, A. I. (1991). Between two cultures: Identity, roles and health. *Healthcare for Women International, 12,* 365–377.

Merrell, J., Kinsella, F., Murphy, F., Philpin, S., & Ali, A. (2005). Support needs of carers of dependent adults from a Bangladeshi community. *Journal of Advanced Nursing, 51,* 549–557.

Mulvihill, M. A., Mailloux, L., & Atkin, W. (2001). *Advancing policy and research responses to immigrant and refugee women's health in Canada.* Ottawa, Canada: Centres of Excellence in Women's Health.

Neufeld, A., Harrison, M. J., Stewart, M. J., Hughes, K., & Spitzer, D. (2002). Immigrant women: Making connections to community resources. *Qualitative Health Research, 12*(6), 752–769.

Ng, R. (1993). Racism, sexism, and immigrant women. In S. Burt, L. Code, & L. Derney (Eds.), *Changing patterns: Women in Canada* (pp. 279–301). Toronto, Canada: McClelland & Stewart.

Pescosolido, B. A. (1986). Migration, medical care preferences and the lay referral system: A network theory of role assimilation. *American Sociological Review, 51,* 523–540.

———. (1991). Illness careers and network ties: A conceptual model of utilization and compliance. *Advances in Medical Sociology, 2,* 161–184.

———. (1992). Beyond rational choice: The social dynamics of how people seek help. *American Journal of Sociology, 97*(4), 1096–1138.

Phillips, M. R. (1993). Strategies used by Chinese families coping with schizophrenia. In D. Davis & S. Harrell (Eds.), *Chinese families in the post-Mao era* (pp. 277–306). Los Angeles: University of California Press.

Remennick, L. I. (1999). Women of the "sandwich" generation and multiple roles: The case of Russian immigrants of the 1990s in Israel. *Sex Roles, 40*(5/6), 347–378.

Rose, D., Carrasco, P., & Charboneau, J. (1998). *The role of "weak ties" in the settlement experience of immigrant women with young children: The case of Central Americans in Montreal* (Working Paper Series 985). Toronto, Canada: Centre of Excellence for Research on Immigration and Settlement. Retrieved March 13, 2002, from http://ceris.metropolis.net

Scharlach, A. E., Kellam, R., Ong, N., Baskin, A., Goldstein, C., & Fox, P. J. (2006). Cultural attitudes and caregiver service use: Lessons from focus groups with racially and ethnically diverse family caregivers. *Journal of Gerontological Social Work, 47,* 133–156.

Simmons, A. B. (1999). Immigration policy: Imagined futures. In S. Halli & L. Driedger (Eds.), *Immigrant Canada: Demographic, economic and social challenges* (pp. 21–50). Toronto, Canada: University of Toronto Press.

Sin, C. H. (2006). Expectations of support among White British and Asian-Indian older people in Britain: The interdependence of formal and informal spheres. *Health and Social Care in the Community, 14,* 215–224.

Slonim-Nevo, V., Cwikel, J., Luski, H., Lankry, M., & Shraga, Y. (1995). Caregiver burden among three-generation immigrant families in Israel. *International Social Work, 38,* 191–204.

Spitzer, D., Neufeld, A., Harrison, M. J., Hughes, K., & Stewart, M. J. (2003). "My wings have been cut, where can I fly?": Gender, migration and caregiving—Chinese and South Asian Canadian perspectives. *Gender and Society, 17*(2), 267–286.

Statistics Canada. (2006). *Women in Canada: A gender-based statistical report* (5th ed., pp. 211–254). Ottawa: Statistics Canada.

Stein, C., Wemmerus, V., Ward, M., Gaines, M., Freeberg, A., & Jewell, T. (1998). "Because they're my parents": An intergenerational study of felt obligation and parental caregiving. *Journal of Marriage & the Family, 60,* 611–622.

Sung, K. T. (1991). Family-centered informal support networks of Korean elderly: The resistance of cultural traditions. *Journal of Cross-Cultural Gerontology, 6*(4), 431–437.

Tabora, B. L., & Flaskerud, J. H. (1997). Mental health beliefs, practices and knowledge of Chinese American immigrant women. *Issues in Mental Health Nursing, 18*(3), 173–189.

Team, V., Markovic, M., & Manderson, L. (2007). Family caregivers: Russian-speaking Australian women's access to welfare support. *Health and Social Care in the Community, 15,* 397–406.

Tirrito, T., & Nathanson, I. (1994). Ethnic differences in caregiving: Adult daughters and elderly mothers. *Affilia, 9*(1), 71–85.

Youn, G., Knight, B., Jeong, H.-S., & Benton, D. (1999). Differences in familialism: Values and caregiving outcomes among Korean, Korean American and White American dementia caregivers. *Psychology and Aging, 14*(3), 355–364.

Yuval-Davis, N. (1997). Ethnicity, gender relations and multiculturalism. In P. Werbner & T. Modood (Eds.), *Debating cultural hybridity: Multi-cultural identities and the politics of anti-racism* (pp. 112–125). London: Zed.

7

Becoming an Advocate in Response to Nonsupportive Interactions

As we indicated in our discussion of family caregivers' perceptions of nonsupportive interactions in Chapter 4, interactions with professional sources of assistance are not always supportive. In our study of women caregivers, we found an unanticipated consequence of the experience of nonsupportive interactions with professionals in the form of advocacy initiatives (Neufeld, Harrison, Stewart, & Hughes, 2008). Some women responded to the negative feelings of lack of trust and powerlessness associated with nonsupportive interactions by becoming strong advocates for their relative and experiencing personal growth in the process. In this chapter, we describe the meaning of advocacy for the women caregivers and the strategies they employed. We also discuss the possibility of advocacy as used by men caregivers.

We use *advocacy* as a term to describe an individual caregiver's proactive response to nonsupportive interactions with professionals in an effort to secure support. Advocacy refers to personal actions and intentions on the part of caregivers to improve the situation of their relative, themselves as caregivers, or others in a similar situation. Our focus is on the individual level of advocacy, although we recognize that advocacy is often used to refer to collective action by groups or organizations (Kar, Pascual, & Chickering, 1999).

Several studies of family caregivers of adults or children and their interactions with professionals have identified the presence of nonsupportive or negative interactions (MaloneBeach & Zarit, 1995; Patterson, Garwick, Bennett, & Blum, 1997; Stadjduhar, 2003), but few have identified caregivers' use of advocacy as a response to these interactions. However, advocacy was identified as a component of ongoing care work in caregiving research with low-income mothers of children with special needs (Litt, 2004). Litt differentiated between direct care work, which incorporated daily, routine assistance, to care of the child and advocacy care work that involved efforts to acquire or fight for resources, correct problems in services available, or engage in extensive negotiations to secure resources. Legault and Ducharme (2009), in a study of daughter caregivers of parents with dementia, described the evolution of the daughter's role as advocate for their parent in long-term care. This role was related to the daughter's evaluation of the quality of care her parent received, as well as her development of trust in the nursing staff and integration into the care setting.

Our specific focus is on a proactive form of advocacy that women caregivers described in response to nonsupportive interactions with professionals. Our research included women in varied situations of providing care for a child (an infant born prematurely or a child with asthma or diabetes) or for an adult (with dementia or cancer). A personal level of advocacy was an important component of their caregiving experience and arose in response to the experience of nonsupportive interactions, which were a catalyst for their advocacy strategies. The advocacy strategies included monitoring, educating, negotiating, and campaigning. As a consequence of their advocacy initiatives, the women experienced personal growth.

As described in Chapter 3, nonsupportive interactions included negative interactions, ineffective interactions, and interactions from which caregivers expected support but from which support was absent (Neufeld, Harrison, Hughes, & Stewart, 2007). Negative interactions with professionals undermined women's credibility as caregivers and included professionals' discounting the issues the women described, minimizing their concerns, misunderstanding what women said, or disbelieving their accounts. More explicit negative actions included blame or criticism, refusal to give support, intimidation of the caregiver, and disrespect. Caregivers' examples of interactions in which the intended aid was ineffective included receiving inadequate information, inappropriate advice, or other offers of aid that they perceived as inadequate despite the potential helper's good intentions. Finally, interactions in which expected support was absent occurred when professionals failed to recognize the women's need for support, there was no potential for support because of conflict, or help was unavailable.

When women experienced these nonsupportive interactions, they reported negative feelings, lack of confidence or trust, lack of power, and a sense that change was hopeless. There were other consequences of the nonsupportive interactions that created challenges to the women's ability to provide care: lack of access to services, diminished options as costs increased, a change in the demands on the caregiver, and concern about future decisions. The women's negative feelings and challenges experienced in the caregiving situation were catalysts for their advocacy intentions and actions.

THE MEANING OF ADVOCACY FOR WOMEN

For women caregivers, the meaning of advocacy included taking charge and persistently asserting oneself as the caregiver with power and rights in a relationship with the health professional. For example, one mother of a child with asthma said:

> That was my first step to asserting myself . . . saying "No, from now on I'm gonna look after this business. I'm not trusting these doctors anymore."

A woman caring for her infant born prematurely said,

> There are those people who just go with the flow. I, on the other hand have to have . . . more input.

A caregiver caring for a relative with dementia referred to

> having to . . . get to the bottom line of something. Telling me half the story is not going to satisfy me.

Or, as another woman caring for a relative with dementia said,

> I have been very vocal, I have not let it go.

Caregivers of adults with cancer sometimes found that they had to establish their positions as caregivers and their right to information about their relative.

The caregiver should also have everything available to them, in order to provide the best possible care, and how can you do that without information?

The constant, invisible, and essential nature of advocacy was evident from the women's descriptions and was associated with an ensuing sense of responsibility and burden. Stress and fatigue often accompanied the women's advocacy efforts. As one mother of a child with diabetes said,

No matter where you go and what you do, it looks really smooth on the surface, but you should see all the treading under water that goes on. It never, ever, ever, ever stops.

Nevertheless, women persisted in their efforts. One young woman caring for her aunt who had cancer described the necessity for advocacy:

You *have* to advocate . . . a lot of it is on you.

She felt that her aunt's health depended on her advocacy.

The feeling of responsibility that's on me . . . it's almost a burden in a sense.

STRATEGIES WOMEN USED IN ADVOCACY

To advocate on behalf of their relatives or themselves or others in a similar situation, women caregivers employed four strategies: monitoring, educating, negotiating, and campaigning.

Monitoring

Monitoring the interactions in their relationships was a process caregivers employed as a basis for sustaining reciprocity in supportive relationships. This type of reciprocity is described in more detail in Chapter 3. As a strategy for advocacy, caregivers used monitoring of their relative's health situation, as well as their relationship with professionals, as a basis for their advocacy initiatives. They monitored their relative's health status, the treatment they received, their response to the interventions of professionals, and the negative characteristics of their environment. Monitoring the caregiving situation included both short-term requirements for monitoring and monitoring that addressed longer-term issues. Short-term monitoring might include assessing daily doses of medication to control the symptoms of asthma, whereas long-term monitoring could include a search for patterns in precipitating factors for a child's acute episodes of asthma. The following quotation illustrates long-term monitoring.

> I've had a daily diary for him . . . we've had to change doctors, and I started going through his diary. . . . He'll [physician] have my notes so he has some idea of what this child has been through. Going through that [diary] I see a pattern here that I never noticed before. (**Mother of a child with asthma**)

A woman living in a rural community, whose adult son was finally diagnosed with cancer after repeated assessments, monitored his weight, pain, and temperature in detail to convince the physicians that their diagnoses of influenza and anorexia were incorrect.

> J. had a high fever . . . he was so sick . . . he's lost more than 35 pounds.

Other caregivers observed interactions and treatments carefully when their relative was hospitalized. One said she learned to say no to the demands of nurses caring for her child.

> No, I will not leave the room when you put the IV in. (**Mother of a child with asthma**)

Another mother said,

> We don't let anything go into her body [daughter with diabetes] unless we know what it is.

Parents whose children had asthma monitored environmental risks in school or office settings and either prevented their children from being exposed to these environments or sought a change in the environment. Monitoring the status of older relatives with dementia was sometimes described as vigilance.

> I became very vigilant . . . to try to protect him for his safety.

On a short-term basis, the mother of one premature infant referred to sitting at the hospital for a good portion of the day to ensure that she could "catch" the physician and get an update on her infant's condition.

Educating

A second advocacy strategy was educating themselves or others such as family members, other caregivers, or professionals. Women caregivers used resources, such as the Internet or courses offered by health care agencies, to inform themselves about their relative's condition and the treatment they needed. A mother of a child with asthma said,

> We had to find out what would work for him. I've had to do the learning on my own.

Examples of educating others included telling other parents and professionals about potential sources of funding for diabetic supplies and coaching other family members of a relative with cancer in how to ask questions to gain the information they needed from physicians. Sometimes women had to educate staff about the best approaches to care.

> He could be tipsy [liable to fall]. I had to remind them that he had to have the raised toilet seat. (**Caregiver of a relative with dementia**)

Women caring for an adult relative with cancer had additional labor in gaining information about their relative's prognosis from physicians. The need to gain further information about their relative's treatment regimen and the associated demands for the caregiver created conflict with physicians, who defined the individual with cancer as the patient and did not necessarily want to respond to the caregiver's questions.

> As a caregiver, there are questions that you need to know, [but] I stopped asking questions because I thought if Mom doesn't want to know the answer, I'm not going to ask . . . . The oncologist only wanted to answer questions that my mom had, because she was the patient. (**Woman caring for a relative with cancer**)

In contrast, health personnel expected mothers of young children to be the primary recipient of information concerning care of a child.

The reluctant response of health and social service professionals to questions of family caregivers of adults may be an unintended consequence of provincial legislation, the Freedom of Information and Protection of Privacy Act (Government of Alberta, 1994), which restricts release of any personal information to another person.

Negotiating

The third strategy of negotiating for change in resources available for their relative has traditionally been associated with advocacy initiatives. Although women sought to negotiate for resources for their relative, often their efforts were described in terms of a struggle to acquire what their relative needed. They often used the analogy of a battle in describing their negotiations to acquire resources. Although the original label for this category was negotiating/fighting, we now consider the term *negotiating* to represent this category adequately.

> I'm pushy. If I have something in my mind I'm going to do it. . . . Some moms don't do that. . . . I think they need to start saying "I'm entitled to that information, that's my right as a mom." (**Mother of an infant born prematurely**)

For mothers of children with asthma or diabetes, there was constant negotiating for financial assistance to ease the costs of care or for their child's special needs to be met within the school.

> It's been a kind of never ending uphill battle, and I went through years of just, what I would call sheer terror, of not knowing what to do. I've been fighting every day, wondering "will this child live through today?" (**Mother of a child with asthma and diabetes**)

Women described how they had to negotiate to get a diagnosis as they tried to convince professionals that something was wrong.

> He [the physician] told me I was being paranoid, that there was nothing wrong with the kid, I just needed to go home and relax. (**Mother of a child with asthma**)

This mother felt that the constant reordering of antibiotics to treat undiagnosed asthma had contributed to her child developing severe allergies that "changed our life totally." She articulated her negotiating role.

> You battle bureaucracy every step of the way. It just doesn't matter whether you're dealing with school or the hospital . . . it robs you of the strength you need.

A woman whose father had dementia described how she had had many battles with the Veteran's Affairs Department but eventually was able to gain helpful assistance.

> They've turned out to be very helpful, but they didn't start out that way. It was, you know, a lot of battles.

The strategy of negotiating became more complex when the care recipient's perspective differed from the caregiver's view. For example, one woman cared for an aunt with cancer who unquestioningly trusted physicians. Although the caregiver thought she would change physicians if she were in a similar situation, she supported her aunt's positive view of her physician and advocated for her in such a way that she [the aunt] would feel more in control of the process.

Campaigning

A fourth advocacy strategy was campaigning. Campaigning was more future-oriented and other-directed than the previous three strategies were. Campaigning frequently was done on behalf of the care recipient and others in similar situations. It sometimes was done to benefit the caregivers themselves. Caregivers wrote letters, developed position statements, and had meetings with key politicians. Other activities used in campaigning included development of a course for other caregivers, adaptation of computer software for pediatric diabetes monitoring, writing books, and establishing a Web site for networking. One mother lobbied the school system for a nurse who could advocate for the family and provide consultation for her daughter and other children within the school setting who had special needs. A woman caring for a relative with cancer described her intention to act for the benefit of other caregivers who might be caught between conflicting policies in different provinces and territories: "I was going to write to the government [regional level of government]."

The mother of an infant born prematurely also described her intent to write to hospitals that had moved her infant twins without notice.

That's where I would write a letter . . . not to be negative, but as a positive; parents should be informed, I think, a minimum of 8 hours before, and 24 would be nice.

One woman campaigned for more family support services at the regional cancer center.

I was going nuts, a lot of the time [and asked] why isn't there a group here, for caregivers? For daughters . . . . The mission statement . . . is all over the place. And it says, "Treat . . . patient and family." And it's not true.

In each caregiving situation, there were women who contacted politicians to make their issues known. A woman caring for her father who had dementia describes her view:

If I have to talk to my MLA [elected Member of the Legislative Assembly], I'll do that . . . because I really felt that I needed to do that. (**Woman caring for a relative with dementia**)

ADVOCACY AND PERSONAL CHANGE

Although there was considerable stress and fatigue in becoming advocates, the women also described the impact of the experience as one of personal growth. They experienced satisfaction when they were able to establish a more egalitarian relationship with health professionals or when they gained understanding of the plight of others. One woman described her increased self-confidence:

I think it's made me a much stronger person . . . . I was very, very, timid.

Another woman identified increased self-awareness:

I've really, really learned a lot about myself. I am determined enough, that . . . if I don't know, I'll go looking for answers.

Women frequently described episodes that revealed how they had become more assertive in communicating with professionals to secure changes that improved care for their relative. For example, a mother of a child with asthma was frustrated with the delays she experienced in emergency when she took her son in during a crisis. Some examples of her comments follow:

> I phoned the hospital and said I'd like to talk to Dr. N. I am starting at the top and working my way down . . . they referred me to . . . a nurse. I said "What I am looking for is some way that when I . . . bring B. in to Emergency they're going to say 'That needs to happen' instead of going though all those steps." They actually implemented a little system . . . . I said "You've admitted him time after time, and while he's laying there gasping, we're going through all the history of my pregnancy." I just wrote it [son's history] out, and I said "Here it is. Put it in the file."

The same mother deliberately sought a younger pediatrician for her son, because she wanted a physician who would be with him throughout his experience. She also became concerned when a physician prescribed a new medication for her son after his second asthma attack. She started the medication but consulted her sister-in-law, who was a pharmacist, and noted that the drug was experimental for children less than 5 years old. The mother described her response as follows:

> It causes heart palpitations, irritability, shakiness . . . and one of the side effects was sudden death . . . If that's even a remote possibility, I am not giving this to my child . . . . I went back to that doctor and said . . . ."I absolutely cannot do this, knowing what the side effects are." . . . After that they didn't give him anything that they didn't explain to me.

A mother who was the sole parent for her diabetic 12-year-old daughter described how she experienced a communication problem with the diabetes clinic where her daughter was seen. She discovered that members of the diabetic team were phoning her daughter while she was at work. Her daughter, who was very guarded about any interaction with a counselor, gave vague responses to questions about checking her blood sugar, such as "I don't remember," "No, maybe," or "I don't think so." The diabetes team assumed the child's behavior was related to high blood sugar levels and left a message on the mother's answering machine requesting that she take time from work to have a special meeting. The mother described her experience:

> I didn't know until then . . . that everybody had been phoning D. D. had been just acting like she was in a daze . . . it was an act. . . . I left that message for the counselor, and then I phoned the nurse, and then I explained to her what

I perceived was going on. And then she explained what they thought was going on. So we managed to communicate and find out what the truth really was. The counselor talked to me after, and they don't call D. anymore.

This mother also described her challenges with interactions with other staff, but particularly the dietician in the clinic:

> The [diabetic] clinic staff didn't understand how hard it is for us . . . until I actually told them what I thought . . . and they've been very understanding since. The dietician was the worst one. She was, oh, it was terrible, condescending, and lecturing. . . . So I finally just explained to her . . . I really told her off. I was very angry . . . and she was very apologetic, 'cause she didn't realize she was doing that.

A woman caring for a relative with cancer who also had diabetes described how she would not take no for an answer and was not willing to be brushed aside without receiving the information she felt she needed.

> I'm going to want to know why you're doing something . . . because I'm looking at the whole picture . . . . The chemo really screws up her diabetes, it really messes with her insulin level . . . so the doctor said "Well, there might be some problems with her insulin level," and I said "What problems am I looking at?" . . . They got me that information.

Another caregiver of a friend with cancer described her perception that the physician communicating her friend's diagnosis was indifferent to the impact of the information. Her friend needed information in response to questions she had come prepared to ask. The caregiver also admired her friend's assertiveness.

> She [the friend] said "Have you ever been faced with a diagnosis like this? . . . You haven't walked down that pathway. And I'm at the door, and you are here with me . . . . You are coming with me down this pathway." He was ready to give her the 20-minute blurb, and she came prepared with questions. The doctor said "You're taking too much time. This is all the time I have." So I said, "When do you have time today? . . . We'll be here at 11 o'clock at night if that works for you . . . G's going to walk out of here having a decision making choice" . . . . We met with him later in the afternoon, and he really shifted. It changed his whole relationship. People at the [hospital] will tell you he is not the same man.

As a consequence of their advocacy efforts, women felt they had more control of the situation, achieved better care for their relative, and were able to relate to health and social service professionals in a more egalitarian partnership role. When positive changes occurred in the quality of care for their relative as a result of their initiatives, they experienced a sense of personal self efficacy and satisfaction.

> I guess I just feel really good about being able to help [their child] as much as I have.

For some women, the experience of nonsupportive interactions and their advocacy efforts also afforded increased understanding of the challenges others faced.

> It's definitely made me more confident and more understanding of other people's plight.

As women experienced positive results and increased confidence through their advocacy efforts, they were able to become more empathic toward others.

MEN CAREGIVERS AND ADVOCACY

Although women were the primary focus of our research on nonsupportive interactions and the response to nonsupport in the form of advocacy, evidence of a similar experience of nonsupportive interactions in our data from research with men caregivers, as outlined in Chapter 3, indicates a need for further study. Similarly, during the review of our published findings and related data from men caregivers, there was evidence of men's use of advocacy strategies such as monitoring and negotiating. For example, a man caring for his wife with Alzheimer's disease experienced difficulty with securing good medical treatment, because he received conflicting diagnoses from different specialists. He later describes how he monitored the situation by keeping a log of his wife's frequent seizures and giving it to her doctor.

> She had been having seizures . . . there was about 45 of them. . . . I kept them all logged . . . and I would give them to the doctor.

The same man sought to help others in a similar situation by becoming active in the Alzheimer's Society and campaigning for more government services.

> I started to get a little more active in the Alzheimer's Society. They've got four subcommittees they've formed to pull information together to make a presentation to the provincial government later this year.

A man caring for his father-in-law talked about negotiating to keep him from being admitted to a mental hospital.

> It's the medical profession that we get into scraps about [laughs], and mainly because they do things and they don't stop to think what effect it's going to have on anybody but themselves. The lady [at the placement agency] [said], "Well, he's just destined for the [mental hospital]." Well, I just blew a top wide open. So we said, "No way." . . . And we're fighting. We were in to see his doctor yesterday.

Another man, who was in business and used to arranging staffing, described how he negotiated with a special care unit that was trying to discharge his wife:

> They kept trying to kick her out, and I wouldn't let them. . . . I knew they had extra staff, and I just fought them all the way.

These descriptions of advocacy initiatives indicate use of similar strategies by men caregivers, but further study is needed to explore in-depth their use of advocacy in response to nonsupportive interactions.

DISCUSSION

A consequence of women's experience of nonsupportive interactions was distress in the form of negative feelings, including lack of trust, and powerlessness, especially when the person for whom they provided care faced deterioration in health and limited access to social services. For some women caregivers, these feelings were the motivation to engage in advocacy strategies, which, when successful in influencing change and generating positive feedback, increased their confidence. They felt good about their own development, exhibiting a psychological level of empowerment that emerged from response to a negative situation (Kar et al., 1999). In this study, distinct from the studies analyzed by Kar and colleagues, the negative situation mobilizing advocacy was nonsupportive interactions with health and social service professionals rather than a form of social oppression, such as problems of violation of human rights, poverty, or abuse. The women's response could be characterized as primarily psychological rather than as a collective, community, or organizational form of empowerment.

Relationships with professionals can be viewed as negotiated exchange relationships (Molm, Peterson, & Takahashi, 1999; Molm, Takahashi, & Peterson, 2000), in which women caregivers seek assistance from more powerful professionals. In this context, the experience of nonsupportive interactions with professionals increased women caregivers' sense of vulnerability and powerlessness and motivated them to engage in advocacy efforts—to strengthen their power base and to facilitate access to needed resources.

This interpretation is supported by other research, which identified the presence of advocacy in response to other caregiving experiences, an increased sense of personal power as a consequence of advocacy, and the negative impact of nonsupportive interactions with professionals that were not accompanied by advocacy. Examples of experiences among women caregivers that contributed to advocacy initiatives included surplus suffering (Clarke & Fletcher, 2004), uncertainty about a child's condition (O'Brien, 2001), adversity (Wuest, 2000), bureaucratic systems (Thorne, 1993), or lack of recognition of the caregiver's competence (MacDonald, 1996). A recurring theme in these examples is the experience of lack of power in their caregiving role, which preceded their advocacy. Increased feelings of powerfulness as a consequence of advocacy initiatives have been reported in other studies with caregivers of adults and children (Rutman, 1996, Thorne, 1993). Successful attempts at advocacy could potentially address women's lack of influence in relationships with professionals and change the basis for negotiated exchange relationships.

A further example of the development of empowerment among caregivers through the process of responding to negative experience is Gibson's (1995) research on empowerment in mothers of chronically ill children. Gibson found that empowerment was a personal process in these mothers that developed in response to frustrations within the family, with the health care system, and with themselves. Some of the mothers' negative experiences with health professionals, particularly physicians, were similar to the nonsupportive interactions identified in our research and included having their concerns minimized, ignored, or negated, as well as receiving prescriptions for medications that did not work as anticipated. Gibson proposed a model of personal empowerment that included critical reflection, taking charge, and holding on, which resulted in women developing "participatory competence," or the ability to advocate for their child. Although Gibson's work supports our finding that the experience of nonsupportive interactions and the accompanying negative feelings were a catalyst for the development of advocacy, her research was limited to mothers caring for a child with neurologic challenges and did not address the specific strategies the women in our studies used.

Other examples include McDonald's (1996) report that mothers of children with asthma became advocates for their child, negotiating for the care the child needed when professionals had discounted the mother's expertise in understanding their child's illness. Wuest (2000) found that women caring for family members in diverse situations used negotiating as the central strategy to address the experience of adversity arising from a demeaning process of seeking help and disillusionment in relationships with health and social service professionals. This response occurred when systems failed to help, provided inadequate help, or made things worse. In a further research example, Pridham (1997) viewed mothers' efforts in seeking help to care for their infant as a personal development outcome of the experience of being a caregiver, and she developed a theoretical model of help-seeking by mothers of young infants based on research.

Our research provided insight into the role of nonsupportive interactions with health and social service professionals as a catalyst for the development of advocacy among women caregivers and identified similar forms of individual-level advocacy initiatives among caregivers in the context of diverse caregiving situations with children and adults. Congruent with the broad context of these findings on advocacy among women caregivers is Carr's (2003) feminist perspective on empowerment practice as a process in which a critical consciousness develops over time and yields a new understanding that becomes the basis for action. Interaction with others in a similar situation facilitates this new understanding and generates possibilities for action as political aspects of their personal situations are identified. The context of women's life experience is influential because they had repeated exposure to difficult situations, such as nonsupportive interactions with professionals, and positive or negative feedback in response to their efforts. Another influential factor in the development of advocacy is education, and women in our study had high levels of education, unlike participants in much of the research exploring experiences of empowerment and advocacy (Carr, 2003; Kar et al., 1999; Litt, 2004).

A key contribution of Carr's (2003) perspective is acknowledgment of the importance of exposure to an originating position that mobilizes a process of empowerment. A distinctive feature of her perspective that is relevant to our study is her view that the basis of powerlessness includes psychological catalysts derived from the absence of external supports, as well as from social or political forms of oppression.

If relationships between family caregivers and professionals are viewed as a form of negotiated exchange relationships (Molm et al., 2000), their experience of dependence and vulnerability in a relationship in which family caregivers hold less power could be heightened by the experience of nonsupportive interactions. This serves as a catalyst to initiate efforts to reduce their dependency and enhance access to resources, a process similar to that interpreted from a critical feminist perspective as a process of empowerment.

Although our research on advocacy as a response to nonsupportive interactions focused on women, we identified examples of similar advocacy initiatives in analysis of our data from men caregivers, but we did not explore differences between men and women. In other research, a study of gender differences among caregivers of a relative with cancer found that men were more likely than women to appraise the caregiving experience as boosting their self esteem (Kim, Baker, & Spillers, 2007). Our research did not specifically address self-esteem, but we did not observe a difference between men and women's descriptions of self-confidence. It is also not known whether the experience of caregiving for a relative with cancer differs from that of caring for a relative with dementia, which was the situation of all of the men in our research, although other research (Kim & Schulz, 2008; Schulz & Sherwood, 2008) has identified that care of relatives with dementia or cancer is challenging in comparison to care of elders with frailty or diabetes. Is the potential for men to receive social rewards and affirmation—for a caregiving role that exceeds the traditional gender expectations—a possible explanation for the finding that men caregivers of a relative with cancer experienced greater self-esteem than women caregivers (Kim et al., 2007)? A study of husbands caring for wives with Alzheimer's disease (Calasanti & King, 2007) found that the men were proud of their ability to complete caregiving tasks and did not worry about their level of proficiency. Some men reported receiving praise from other women, who noted that few men would do this kind of work, whereas the men observed that similar comments were not made to women caregivers because they were expected to give care.

Another unanswered question is whether men who engaged in advocacy initiatives were demonstrating a behavior and confidence level consistent with their past employment and personal life experience as men, or whether these initiatives represented development of a new level of confidence and sense of empowerment. One qualitative study of sons caring for a parent with dementia (Campbell & Carroll, 2007) reported that sons took an attitude toward caregiving of just doing whatever was necessary, which may reflect a carryover of a "take charge" attitude that is stereotypically masculine in North American culture. Further research is needed with men caregivers to explore the meaning of advocacy in response to nonsupportive interactions in-depth and whether the experience of engaging in these initiatives is a source of increasing self-confidence or growth for men.

Research with men caregivers and analysis of possible gender differences among caregivers in the experience of the support process, including nonsupportive interactions, is a necessary foundation for delivery of gender sensitive care. Miers (2002) contends that a gender-sensitive approach in research identifies regularities among men and women, while attending to particulars in the situation, and avoids universalizing the views of men or women. She suggests that attention to the specific context within which men and women provide care includes identification of the sociopolitical context within which men and women differentially experience links between public expectations and private care or with cultural stereotypes about aging as well as gender.

Initially research on family caregiving focused on women caregivers, based on the assumption that women were the main family caregivers and that, if men did take on a caregiving role, they were more likely than women to seek support from sources outside the family (Kaye & Applegate, 1995). More recently, there has been increased awareness of the number of men, particularly spouses, who are family caregivers, and an effort has been made to conduct gender-sensitive research on family caregiving.

The assumption that women provided care in the home also influenced research done on parenting and early childhood development, which initially focused on mother-child relationships but now is examining the importance of fathering to child development (Day & Lamb,

2004; Pruett, 1998). Russell's (2004) finding of the co-existence of men caregivers' performance of nurturing and management skills and the finding by Calasanti and Bowen (2006) that men and women both cross gender boundaries—that they established in early marriage to do care work for their spouse—provide evidence of the importance of gender-sensitive approaches to research and the limitations of stereotypes of men's caregiving roles.

In summary, our research on the meaning and development of advocacy as a response of family caregivers to nonsupportive interactions with professionals contributes useful insight into their experience. Our findings suggest the potential for emergence of an individual level of advocacy to be a mechanism for empowerment, especially for women, interacting with professionals in a form of negotiated exchange relationship. We suggest the need for further research to address advocacy among men caregivers experiencing nonsupportive interactions to facilitate gender-sensitive approaches to research and practice with family caregivers.

NOTE

The data reported in this chapter were drawn from a study of nonsupportive interactions of women caregivers in four caregiving situations that was reported in Neufeld, Harrison, Stewart, and Hughes (2008).

REFERENCES

Calasanti, T., & Bowen, M. E. (2006). Spousal caregiving and crossing gender boundaries: Maintaining gendered identities. *Journal of Aging Studies, 20*, 253–263.

Calasanti, T., & King, N. (2007). Taking "women's work" "like a man": Husbands' experiences of care work. *The Gerontologist, 47*(4), 516–527.

Campbell, L., & Carroll, M. (2007). The incomplete revolution: Theorizing gender when studying men who provide care to aging parents. *Men and Masculinities, 9*(4), 491–508.

Carr, E. S. (2003). Rethinking empowerment theory using a feminist lens: The importance of process. *Affilia, 18*(1), 8–20.

Clarke, J., & Fletcher, P. (2004). Parents as advocates: Stories of surplus suffering when a child is diagnosed and treated for cancer. *Social Work and Health Care, 39*, 107–127.

Day, R. D., & Lamb, M. E. (Eds.). (2004). *Conceptualizing and measuring father involvement*. Mahwah, NJ: Erlbaum.

Gibson, C. H. (1995). The process of empowerment in mothers of chronically ill children. *Journal of Advanced Nursing, 21*, 1201–1210.

Government of Alberta. (1994). Freedom of Information and Protection of Privacy Act. Retrieved June 27, 2007, from http://foip.gov.ab.ca

Kar, S. B., Pascual, C. A., & Chickering, K. L. (1999). Empowerment of women for health promotion: A meta-analysis. *Social Science & Medicine, 49*, 1431–1360.

Kaye, L. W. & Applegate, J. S. (1995). Men's style of nurturing elders. In D. Sabo & D. F. Gordon (Eds.), *Men's health and illness: Gender, power and the body* (pp. 205–221). Thousand Oaks, CA: Sage.

Kim, Y., Baker, F., & Spillers, R. L. (2007). Cancer caregivers' quality of life: Effects of gender, relationship and appraisal. *Journal of Pain and Symptom Management, 34*(3), 294–304.

Kim, Y., & Schulz, R. (2008). Family caregivers' strains: Comparative analysis of cancer caregiving with dementia, diabetes, and frail elder caregiving. *Journal of Aging and Health, 20*(5), 483–503.

Legault, A. & Ducharme, F. (2009). Advocating for a parent with dementia in a long-term care facility. *Journal of Family Nursing, 15*, 198–219.

Litt, J. (2004). Women's carework in low-income households: The special case of children with attention deficit hyperactivity disorder. *Gender & Society, 18*, 625–644.

MacDonald, H. (1996). Mastering uncertainty: Mothering the child with asthma. *Pediatric Nursing, 22*, 55–64.

MaloneBeach, E., & Zarit, S. (1995). Dimensions of social support and social conflict as predictors of caregiver depression. *International Psychogeriatrics, 7*(1), 25–38.

Miers, M. (2002). Developing an understanding of gender sensitive care: Exploring concepts and knowledge. *Journal of Advanced Nursing, 40*(1), 69–77.

Molm, L., Peterson, G., & Takahashi, N. (1999). Power in negotiated and reciprocal exchange. *American Sociological Review, 64*, 876–890.

Molm, L., Takahashi, N., & Peterson, G (2000). Risk and trust in social exchange: An experimental test of a classical proposition. *American Journal of Sociology, 105*(5), 1396–1427.

Neufeld, A., Harrison, M. J., Hughes, K., & Stewart, M. (2007). Non-supportive interactions in the experience of women family caregivers. *Health and Social Care in the Community, 15*(6), 530–541.

Neufeld, A., Harrison, M. J., Stewart, M., & Hughes, K. (2008). Advocacy of women family caregivers: Response to nonsupportive interactions with professionals. *Qualitative Health Research, 18*(3), 301–310.

O'Brien, M. E. (2001). Living in a house of cards: Family experiences with long-term childhood technology dependence. *Journal of Pediatric Nursing, 16*, 13–22.

Patterson, J., Garwick, A., Bennett, F., & Blum, R. (1997). Social support in families of children with chronic conditions: Supportive and nonsupportive behaviours. *Developmental and Behavioral Pediatrics, 18*(6), 383–391.

Pridham, K. F. (1997). Mothers' help seeking as care initiated in a social context. *Image: Journal of Nursing Scholarship, 29*(1), 65–70.

Pruett, K. D. (1998). Role of the father. *Pediatrics, 102*(5, Suppl. E), 1253–1261.

Russell, R. (2004). Social networks among elderly men caregivers. *Journal of Men's Studies, 13*(1), 121–142.

Rutman, D. (1996). Caregiving as women's work: Women's experiences of powerfulness and powerlessness as caregivers. *Qualitative Health Research, 6*, 90–111.

Schulz, R., & Sherwood, P. (2008). Physical and mental health effects of family caregiving. *American Journal of Nursing, 108*(9), 23–27.

Stajduhar, K. I. (2003). Examining the perspectives of family members involved in the delivery of palliative care at home. *Journal of Palliative Care, 19*(1), 27–35.

Thorne, S. E. (1993). *Negotiating health care: The social context of chronic illness.* Newbury Park, CA: Sage.

Wuest, J. (2000). Negotiating with helping systems: An example of grounded theory evolving through emergent fit. *Qualitative Health Research, 10,* 51–70.

8   A Guide to Support Facilitation

In this chapter we integrate the dimensions of the support process and the experiences of family caregivers that we presented in earlier chapters and discuss how our research findings have potential for use in clinical practice. In agreement with others (Barbour, 2000; Kearney, 2001; Morse, Hutchinson, & Penrod, 1998; Sandelowski, 1997, 2004) we contend that sound qualitative research findings have utility for practice in health care settings. Kearney provides a framework for the utilization of qualitative research findings that are rich in complexity and discovery and that fit with the clinical issues faced by professionals. This framework lists four ways that qualitative research findings can provide guidance to practice and appears to be an appropriate fit with our research program. Findings can facilitate insight or empathy for patients or families who share the experience described in the qualitative research, provide guidance in the assessment of status or progress in an individual's response to a health problem, give direction to professionals in how to assist patients and their families through anticipatory guidance, and provide suggestions on how professionals could coach patients and families in responses to their situation.

We begin this chapter by presenting an integration of the dimensions of the support process derived from our research on the experiences of family caregivers. We then discuss ways that our findings have potential for use in clinical practice. Finally, the reader is invited to examine the utility of our framework through consideration of suggested guiding questions and three family caregiving scenarios with accompanying eco-maps that reflect the populations that were included in our research.

CAREGIVERS' EXPERIENCE OF THE SUPPORT PROCESS

An overview of the dimensions of the support process derived from all our studies of family caregivers was presented in Figure 1.4 in Chapter 1. The overview included personal and social influencing factors, the processes of monitoring, reflecting, and mobilizing support; and the perception of the caregiver that interactions with others were supportive or nonsupportive. Several consequences of the support experience were identified. We suggest that an understanding of these situational and personal dimensions can inform the ways in which professionals approach support facilitation with family caregivers. For ease of presentation, we do not repeat here the specific studies from which each component of the framework was derived, as these were identified in Chapters 2 through 7, and a summary of participants in each study was included in Table 1.1 in Chapter 1.

Influencing Factors

Initially we consider personal and social factors in the caregiving situation that may influence the mobilization of support by family caregivers. These are presented in detail in Figure 8.1.

The inner circle in Figure 8.1 represents the personal characteristics of the family caregiver that were influential in their experience of support. These include the caregiver's personal and cultural beliefs and expectations, their family role, caregiving goals, ability to monitor and reflect on their situation, and their communication skills including language or languages that they speak. For example, the cultural beliefs and personal expectations for caregiving for one caregiver may include a belief in filial responsibility and expectations for family obligations, whereas another caregiver may value independence and place a priority on reciprocity in relationships. Expectations for their family role as spouse, son, or daughter might reflect cultural and societal values and influence their choices and goals as caregivers. Caregivers motivated by beliefs about reciprocity considered the time frame in their relationships. Caregivers for elders often considered a long history and the contributions of the care recipient in the distant past, whereas mothers of

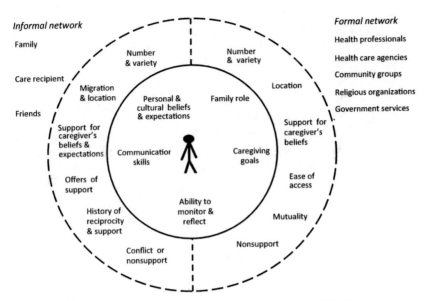

Figure 8.1. Personal and social factors influencing a caregiver's mobilization of support from his or her social networks.

infants born prematurely held future-oriented expectations for reciprocity. Other caregivers, including subgroups of men and women caring for an older relative with dementia, mothers of infants born prematurely, and immigrant women caregivers, described their motivation for caregiving in terms of obligation to the relationship. These beliefs reflected their commitment to responsibilities assumed in marital and family relationships and were reinforced by cultural expectations.

As suggested in our analysis, these beliefs may be embedded in broader commitments to justice or caring that reflect societal values. In the context of immigrant women's experience, beliefs about obligations to care were embedded in cultural expectations of their familial roles as well as their role as women in preserving and communicating cultural beliefs, particularly following immigration. The ability to communicate was identified as an important skill in mobilizing support, which might be limited by lack of facility in English for immigrant caregivers. Other caregivers were hesitant to make verbal requests for support and relied on nonverbal cues that indicated their need for assistance. The ability of caregivers to monitor and reflect on their situation was also an important influence on support mobilization and is addressed later in this chapter in relation to processes of monitoring, reflecting, and mobilizing support.

In the broken outer circle in Figure 8.1, we represent the interaction of family caregivers with their informal networks of family, care recipient, and friends (on the left side of the diagram) as well as the formal social network of professionals and programs, including health and social service professionals, health care agencies, community groups, religious organizations, and government services (on the right). As our findings indicated, the number and variety of informal network members (composition), experience of migration and the location of network members, the support they provide for the caregiver's values, their willingness to offer support, and their history of reciprocal and supportive or conflicted and nonsupportive interactions were influential in how the caregiver was able to mobilize support. Caregivers who had more diverse networks expressed the greatest satisfaction and received the most frequent and broadest range of support. Caregivers in kin-dominated networks experienced more conflict. Some caregivers were socially isolated, with small networks that sometimes comprised primarily professionals. Immigrant caregivers often reported small social networks and a loss of support from family and friends because of their migration to another country.

Beliefs about reciprocity and obligation were influential in the caregivers' perceptions of relationships with family and friends in the informal social network. Reciprocal relationships were characterized by a history of positive interactions or the expectation of positive interaction in the future, attributions of an intent to convey positive responses (e.g., in relationships with the care recipient), the waiving or suspension of expectations for reciprocity, or an altruistic view that assistance could be passed on to others and not necessarily exchanged within the same relationship. For many family caregivers, their relationship with the care recipient was an important influence on the process of mobilizing support. Some care recipients were able to reciprocate support through positive comments or had a history of providing support to the caregiver. Caregivers who reported conflict or nonsupport in their interactions with family and friends faced barriers to mobilizing support.

Among members of the formal social network we include health professionals, health care agencies, community groups, religious organizations, and government services. Mobilization of support from professional sources, similar to the informal network, was also influenced by the number and variety of professional sources with ties to the caregiver, their location, the support they provided for the caregivers' beliefs, policies affecting ease of access and available resources, mutuality in interactions between the family caregiver and professionals, and whether caregivers perceived their interactions with representatives of the formal network as nonsupportive. For example, delivery of services in a rushed manner without consultation with the caregiver created challenges. Policies that limited access, poor coordination of professional services, high cost of services, the lack of suitable facilities or programs, and decisions about the care of their family member made unilaterally by health care staff were key barriers to the caregiver's experience of support.

Processes of Monitoring, Reflecting, and Mobilizing of Support

Within the context of support mobilization, caregivers monitored the caregiving situation, reflected on their interactions with family, friends, and professionals, and engaged in decisions and actions to mobilize and use support. The relationship of monitoring and reflection to the mobilization and use of support or the choice to go it alone is addressed in Figure 8.2.

In monitoring their caregiving situations, family caregivers vigilantly observed the health status and needs of their relatives. These observations were planned, systematic, and conducted over time as caregivers sought to identify the care recipient's needs and changes in their

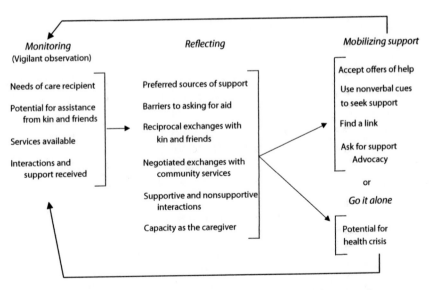

Figure 8.2. Relationships of monitoring and reflecting and mobilizing support.

health status. Included in the caregivers' observations were the nonverbal responses of the care recipient. The caregivers also monitored the potential for assistance within their relationships with family and friends and the professional services available in their community, as well as the nature of their interactions with and support received from others.

In reflecting on their observations, caregivers considered their beliefs about the preferred sources of support and barriers to asking for aid. Barriers and risks associated with making a request for assistance included the loss of privacy, the potential for refusal of assistance, and the time and effort needed to coach others to provide assistance. Family caregivers reflected on their experience of past and ongoing reciprocal, supportive exchanges with family and friends, and the nature of and mutuality in negotiated exchanges with community resources. Other considerations were their perceptions of supportive and nonsupportive interactions, and their personal capacity as a caregiver, including whether they had the physical and emotional resources to continue to provide care. Caregivers who used support sought to mobilize support from family and friends or professional sources by accepting offers of help. Caregivers expressed a strong preference for accepting offers of assistance from others rather than directly asking for support. Some caregivers were unable to ask for support, even when they wanted assistance and demonstrated their need through the use of nonverbal cues, although these were not always recognized. They sought to locate a knowledgeable person who could be a link to a source of aid. If they faced the need to make a specific request for support, they preferred to use support from family and friends, those with whom they had exchanged support, or with whom there was the potential for reciprocity in the future. In mobilizing support from the formal network, caregivers weighed the psychosocial costs of negotiating access to services with professionals in relation to their personal goals in caregiving, the behaviors that they might encounter from professionals that would facilitate or impede their ability to secure aid, and the possibility of mutuality in decision making. In some situations, caregivers engaged in advocacy initiatives for their relative to secure adequate assistance.

Alternatively, some caregivers continued to provide by length care alone without accepting assistance, and resisted seeking aid. In some situations, caregivers delayed seeking assistance until a crisis occurred that precipitated mobilization of support. In response to a crisis, they chose to give up their independence, opened the door to the possibility of accepting help, and sought resources that were a good match for their relative and their caregiving situation. Once assistance was secured, the iterative cycle of monitoring, reflecting, and mobilizing support continued. The processes of monitoring and reflecting were iterative and ongoing, as indicated by the arrows in Figure 8.2.

Many of the elements of caregivers' experience of support identified in our research were also reported in a literature review of dyadic support within intimate, couple relationships. Using a perspective of dyadic stress and coping, Rafaeli and Gleason (2009) identified from the literature several ways in which support can be skillful in achieving intended goals, rather than unskillful and associated with unwelcome costs. They proposed a model of the support process that addresses: development over time including the stages of identifying need, appraisal and communication, and action; multiple dimensions of need and support provision with optimal matching; and equity in reciprocal exchange of support. Findings of our research also revealed changing caregiving requirements over time, barriers, preferences and issues associated with appraisal and requests for support, challenges in securing matching resources, the threat to self-esteem of being explicitly indebted to others, and the impact of reciprocity and equity in relationships with friends and family or professionals. Like Rafaeli and Gleason, we suggest that many of the negative effects of support initiatives can be addressed, and support provided more skillfully when these dimensions are considered and enhanced.

IMPLICATIONS OF THE SUPPORT PROCESS FOR PRACTICE INTERVENTIONS

The four modes of clinical application of qualitative research findings proposed by Kearney (2001) can be used to discuss potential ways that our research can inform clinical practice and facilitate support to family caregivers. These modes of clinical application (insight or empathy, assessment of status or progress, anticipatory guidance, and coaching) vary in their degree of visibility and patient involvement. For example, our research findings can contribute to clinicians' insight and ability to understand the experience of a family caregiver, the differing perspectives that caregivers may hold about their goals in giving care, and the common factors that influence their choices in mobilizing support. We learned in our research that the interpretation of an action as supportive or nonsupportive was particular to an individual family caregiver.

Dynamics of a specific caregiver's situation may be better understood when professionals recognize that the same action, intended to be supportive, can been seen as either supportive or nonsupportive depending on the specific caregiver and situation. A clinician who was aware of this finding might decide to explore with family caregivers how they view the actions of others in their network and whether those actions are seen as supportive

Knowledge of the range of dimensions of social support and the characteristics of social networks as documented in our research could foster increased detail in assessment of the support available to family caregivers. Professional assessments may become more detailed by incorporating information about the factors such as personal, societal, and cultural beliefs and expectations that influence the choices a caregiver makes. Use of a detailed method of documenting the social network of a caregiver, such as ecomaps, can highlight current sources of support, gaps in support available, and areas of potential for assistance from programs and policies or family and friends.

Anticipatory guidance and coaching are modes of application of qualitative research findings that involve clients more directly than either enhanced professional insight or more detailed assessment. We suggest that the findings from our research have potential in the area of anticipatory guidance for caregivers. Many caregivers feel alone in their situation and search for information about the expected course of events in situations similar to their own. Exposure to information generated in qualitative research about the varied experience of other caregivers can assist an individual family caregiver to anticipate possible challenges and consider potential resources.

Coaching, the final form of application of qualitative research findings to practice suggested by Kearney (2001), also may be relevant. For example, a health professional may facilitate a caregiver's ability to sustain reciprocity and constructed reciprocity in relationships and to overcome cognitive and situational barriers to asking for assistance. Consideration of the components of the process of support mobilization in relation to kin and friends or professional sources can expand practitioners' knowledge of possibilities for clinical exploration and ability to coach caregivers as they work through the process of mobilizing aid. Questions posed by health care workers to a family caregiver about support he or she used or provided in the past may help a caregiver recognize an individual or an agency that would be a potential source of assistance for the current situation.

Hooyman and Gonyea (1999) argue that interventions that focus on individual change, such as assisting individuals to cope or adjust to their situation, may not improve their lives if structural causes for the stress on family caregivers, such as the lack of home care services in a community or decreased funding for adult day programs, are not examined. The importance of structural or "upstream" social conditions that influence the individual's experience of support has also been stressed by Berkman and colleagues (Berkman, Glass, Brissette, & Seeman, 2000). The framework provided by Kearney (2001) focuses on the role of nurses working with an individual client and does not directly address the issue of structural or social conditions. There are, however, opportunities for interventions that influence structural conditions. Nurses and other health professionals, particularly those practitioners who work in the community or who have administrative positions, may have influence on agency, public and social policy, and the development or maintenance of programs for family caregivers when they participate on social planning committees and interface with government or other funders of health and social programs. Individual practitioners may also address structural conditions that affect family caregivers when they advocate on behalf of their clients and family caregivers in obtaining access to services. Examples of this role from our research include professionals who advocated for parents seeking financial support for the cost of diabetic supplies for their daughter and others who supported the appeal of an immigrant mother to have her child admitted to a rehabilitative service for children with developmental delays.

Our findings on the importance of mutuality between family caregivers and health professionals in planning and providing care to a family member and the impact of mutuality on support for the family caregiver have important implications for the manner in which health professionals carry out interventions. The inherent imbalance of power between family caregivers and health care professionals is similar to that between professionals and many clients. The need to recognize the knowledge and skills of families and care recipients, and the need for partnerships or collaborations based on mutuality have been stressed by others (Eisner & Wright, 1986; Hooyman & Gonyea, 1999; Legault & Ducharme, 2009; Rafaeli & Gleason, 2009). Our research suggests that if the relationship between nurse or other professional and caregiver is based on mutuality with recognition of the experience and goals of the family caregiver, then the assessment of their concerns and interventions that provide anticipatory guidance or coaching may be more acceptable to the caregiver.

Rafaeli and Gleason (2009), in the context of research on intimate couple relationships, suggest that the provision of support in an indirect manner that makes support provision less visible to the recipient, is less costly and more acceptable to the recipient, as it reduces indebtedness. Our research examined the experience of family caregivers and did not address the intentions of health professionals or their choice of methods in providing support. A query for future research is whether direct and indirect support have different outcomes for family caregivers and whether indirect support may be acceptable to those caregivers who choose to go it alone in caregiving.

Ultimately, the professional's reflective clinical judgment establishes the fit of credible research findings with a specific caregiving situation. We do not address here the criteria for establishing credibility of qualitative research, such as those used in the process of peer review for publication, but suggest that the reader consult one of the many available qualitative research texts for background in this area. In the context of credible research findings, we encourage clinicians to use their experiential knowledge as a basis to consider the following questions and the potential fit with their practice.

QUESTIONS TO CONSIDER ABOUT CAREGIVERS' EXPERIENCE OF SUPPORT

Using an approach similar to that of Morse, Hutchinson, and Penrod (1998), we present a series of questions for exploration in relation to the components of the proposed framework. Consideration of the questions is intended to facilitate insight into individual circumstances and behavior and to enable the health professional to provide appropriate care. The purpose of the questions is to promote critical thinking and reflection by practitioners, and not to impose a rigid pattern for care. For ease of linkage to the framework, we have inserted prior to each set of questions the key framework headings from Figure 1.4 in Chapter 1, "Caregivers' Experience of Social Support" (p.19).

Personal and Social Influencing Factors

1. What personal, social, or cultural beliefs and/or expectations and what family role does the caregiver hold?
2. What are his or her goals in caregiving?

3. How would you describe the caregiver's social network, including family, friends, professionals, and community programs in terms of number, variety, location, support for the caregiver, and history of reciprocity and conflict, as well as recent or expected changes?

4. What are the care recipient's expectations of members of his or her social network, and what support, if any, do they give the caregiver?

Monitoring and Reflecting

1. How does the caregiver assess his or her situation in terms of caregiving demands, his or her relative's current and expected health status, and his or her own ability to continue to give care?

2. What is the caregiver's experience of supportive or nonsupportive interactions with kin, friends, and community services, and what potential sources of additional support might be explored?

Mobilizing Support

1. What are the caregiver's preferences in receiving support in terms of desired sources or the choice to provide caregiving alone?

2. How does the caregiver express a need for support? How have these efforts been successful?

3. What does the caregiver consider when making requests for support from kin and friends or professional sources (e.g., reciprocity, barriers)?

4. What professional or community resources are known and/or sought? How will the caregiver initiate contact (or how was contact initiated in the past)?

Perception of Supportive and Nonsupportive Interactions

1. How does the caregiver describe the interactions that he or she has with kin, friends, and professionals? In what ways does the caregiver perceive them as supportive or nonsupportive?

2. What are the caregiver's perceptions of the potential to modify nonsupportive interactions and/or foster supportive, reciprocal, or mutual interactions?

Caregiver Consequences

1. What are the caregiver's feelings about him- or herself and the support that he or she receives in the caregiving situation?
2. In what ways (if any) has the caregiver revised his or her expectations of others or of him- or herself in the caregiving role?
3. How (if at all) has the caregiver become an advocate or experienced personal growth in his or her role?
4. How has the caregiver's experience of support while caregiving affected his or her social network or relationships?

Professional Perspective

1. From your perspective as a professional, what potential additional support resources are needed and/or available?
2. What additional potential sources of aid could the caregiver consider among family and friends?
3. What additional potential resources are available in the community? Given the specific characteristics of this caregiving situation and community resources, what considerations are important for support mobilization initiatives?
4. How would you work toward mutuality in your contacts with the family caregiver?
5. How would your actions be nondirective or directive?
6. Within your professional role and agency mandate, what resources and options are available? What opportunities exist to influence agency, public, or social policy to improve resources and options for caregivers in this situation?

CAREGIVING SCENARIOS

We invite the reader to consider three scenarios in relation to the findings of our research on family caregiving and support and the guiding questions presented in the previous section. Although we recognize that the information included in each scenario is brief, it provides a beginning for discussion of the use of our findings in practice. The composite scenarios and accompanying ecomaps were constructed from our research, and depict family caregivers' experience of social support in different caregiving situations. For each caregiving scenario and accompanying ecomap, we pose sample questions that a health professional might ask in gathering more information about the client to guide interventions.

Ecomaps, originally developed for use in practice, are a graphic portrayal of the social network and identify key sources of support including connections with kin, friends, employers, professionals, and affiliations or club memberships (Wright & Leahy, 2005). Ecomaps can be a useful tool for practitioners, as the process of developing an ecomap facilitates detailed discussion of caregivers' connections with others. They are also useful catalysts to assist caregivers in reflecting on their own social network. Although we discuss the use of ecomaps in our research in more detail in Chapter 9, a brief description is included here to outline their use as an aid for practitioners in assessing and documenting the nature of caregivers' social networks.

The ecomaps in Figures 8.3, 8.4, and 8.5 represent the social network described for each caregiver in the accompanying composite scenario. Each circle placed on a caregiver's ecomap represents a relationship that influenced the caregiver's experience of support while caregiving. We depict the nature of the relationship, including the dimensions of energy flow (i.e., reciprocal or one-way exchanges), intensity (multiple lines), and stress or conflict (cross-hatched lines). Broken lines are used to depict tenuous relationships and support sources. In these illustrations, we include potential sources of support to be explored, although social connections are not yet established, as well as connections that are no longer available (e.g., deceased).

Dementia Caregiving Situation

[Figure 8.3] Since Rose retired five years ago, she has cared for her husband, Ron, who has advanced Alzheimer's disease. Ron can no longer dress or wash himself, needs constant reminding to eat at mealtimes, and has wandered out of the house twice in the last month. Rose and Ron have three grown daughters, who live nearby but rarely come to visit. One daughter has two preschool-aged children. The daughters feel that their mother is not doing enough for their dad, and they do not want to hear her talk about her caregiving. They feel that going to the day program every day is too much for their father. "He needs time at home," they argue. "No wonder he's so forgetful. You're always sending him off to spend his days with strangers." Rose has never done well with conflict. She has not confronted her daughters with how hurt she is by their comments.

Rose does talk with the staff at the center and feels they understand how demanding Ron's care is and how much Rose needs monthly overnight respite to get caught up on her sleep. Weekly letters from her sister in another city also comfort Rose. Her sister cared for their mother for many years and understands how hard it can get. Alana, from next door, brings Rose and Ron a hot meal once a week. She helped find Ron the last time he wandered away from the house. When Alana's children were young, Rose used to babysit for her.

The social worker at the day program has started looking into nursing homes for Ron as Rose's back is bothering her more and more from helping Ron in and out of the bathtub. Location, expense, and Ron's eligibility for veteran benefits need consideration. There is a veterans' facility in the neighborhood, but so far Rose has not been able to get the documentation needed from Veterans Affairs so that Ron can qualify for the subsidy.

Rose has days when she feels angry at her children, sad about not seeing her grandchildren, guilty that she is not doing enough for Ron, and worried about the finances. "I must be overtired," she then says to herself, and phones Veterans Affairs yet again.

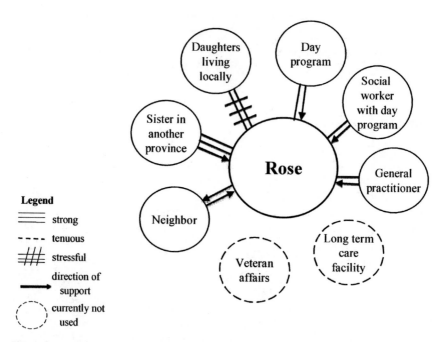

Figure 8.3. Ecomap of supportive and nonsupportive interactions for Rose.

We illustrate three of the questions we posed for exploration of social support from this scenario. What is the caregiver's experience of supportive or nonsupportive interactions with kin, friends, and community services, and what potential sources of additional support might be explored? What are the caregiver's feelings about her experience of social support in her caregiving situation? What does she consider in making requests for support from kin and friends or professional sources (e.g., reciprocity, barriers)?

Rose is experiencing nonsupportive interactions with family members (depicted as hatched lines on the ecomap) and consequently is experiencing negative, hurt feelings. She is hesitant to disclose her feelings to her daughters. In mobilizing support, she is comfortable accepting help from her neighbor, whom she has assisted in the past and has known for a long time. The two-way arrows between Rose and her neighbor show the history of reciprocity between them. Her link to professional sources of assistance is the social worker at the adult day program that her husband attends, and this link may assist her in securing a placement for Ron.

With this information, the social worker working with Rose would be aware of the importance of listening to Rose describe her disappointment in the nonsupport from her daughters and the need to assist Rose in her communications with Veterans Affairs. The staff in the day care program could also explore with Rose some ways to help her to communicate with her daughters about her stress and her need for more relief from caregiving. They might also explore with Rose other relationships in which she has a history of reciprocal support and from whom she might be able to seek some assistance.

Mother Caring for an Infant Born Prematurely

[Figure 8.4] Katia had been married for 12 years when, on her 34th birthday, she gave birth to Michael, her first baby, 7 weeks early. She and her husband had never planned to have children, but when Katia's sisters started having children, Katia changed her mind. Her husband reluctantly agreed to "try for one."

Michael has been home from the hospital for a week now, and Katia is exhausted. As much as she tried to breastfeed Michael in the hospital, the nurses said that tube feeds were the only way to get the weight on. Often they would do the tube feed without even giving Katia a chance to breastfeed. Sometimes they would even forget to give him the breast milk that

Katia had expressed for him. Katia is very relieved to have Michael home, but her sisters' offers to come and help with the baby so that Katia can get some rest have not materialized. Katia had been pleased with their offers, as she is hesitant to ask for help. Although her husband showed some delight with his baby son, he made it clear that it was not his idea to have a baby, so he would not be getting up at night. Besides, he is anxious about his new job and needs support from Katia while he adjusts.

The public health nurse is Katia's lifeline. She has nothing but praise for Katia's persistent efforts with breastfeeding. She is a fountain of baby information and has given Katia some names of moms in the neighborhood who hosted a play group for mothers and babies.

Katia's godmother phones just about every day to ask about Michael and to listen to Katia's concerns. She even arranged for the women at her church to bring over meals for a few weeks.

Katia's situation can demonstrate the utility of other guiding questions. What are the caregiver's preferences in receiving support in terms of desired sources or a choice to provide caregiving alone? What professional or community resources are known and/or sought?

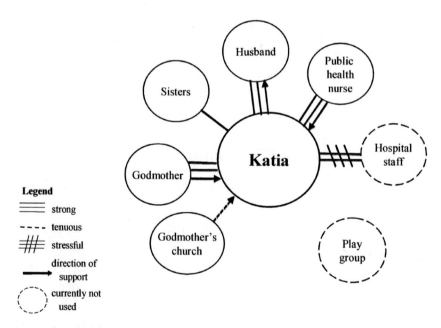

Figure 8.4. Ecomap of supportive and nonsupportive interactions for Katia.

Katia's preferred source of support is her family, especially her sisters, who had volunteered their assistance with the baby prior to his birth. The ecomap shows a tenuous single line between Katia and her sisters, indicating the limited contact she now has. Her husband is seeking her support to adjust to a new job and does not provide support to Katia with the new baby (the arrow on the ecomap shows support provided to the husband and none received from him in caring for Michael). Katia's godmother is supportive and may be a continuing source of support in the future.

In terms of professional resources, the public health nurse is viewed by Katia as supportive and is her potential link to outside sources of support from the community, which might include a neighborhood play group with new mothers. As a professional the public health nurse might continue to explore other questions with Katia. How does Katia express her need for support? Did she ask her sisters for assistance, or does she expect that they will offer help without being asked? In what ways has there been reciprocal support between the sisters in the past? Does Katia see the meals provided by the women at her godmother's church as a supportive action? What potential is there for continued contact with these women, and is there any likelihood of future emotional support? Would Katia consider attending a play group for new mothers and babies in her neighborhood? The public health nurse could share educational resources with Katia, such as parenting books or videotapes that include concerns of new fathers, which might be of interest to her husband as he becomes more comfortable in his new job. Providing education to all family members is one way that health professionals can assist family caregivers (Hooyman & Gonyea, 1999) as informed family members are more likely to be able to provide some support to the family caregiver when they become more aware of the concerns of others and their own questions and concerns are addressed.

Immigrant Woman Caring for a Child

[Figure 8.5] Saleema came from India six years ago. She speaks Punjabi, is a widow, and has a daughter in first grade. She was sponsored by her brother to come to Canada. Both Saleema and her brother live in an area in which many others live who immigrated from India. Saleema is taking care of her daughter, who is identified as being developmentally delayed. Her daughter requires extra assistance, and the school provided a part-time aide to help her. Saleema feels that the care she gives is important to help her daughter improve. Because she cannot speak any English, Saleema feels cut off from the school and from health care in Canada. She believes that her daughter could get better care if she knew what services were available in her area. At present, Saleema relies on her brother to act as her interpreter in contacts with English-speaking agencies.

Questions about factors influencing the support process and the caregivers' assessment of the need for support are especially important for Saleema. What personal, social, or cultural beliefs and/or expectations does the caregiver hold? What are her caregiving goals? How does she express a need for support? What does she consider in making requests for support from kin and friends or professional sources (e.g., reciprocity, barriers)? What was Saleema's experience in her contact with the school and with the professionals who conducted the developmental assessment?

Several influencing factors are important for Saleema as she seeks to care for her daughter with special needs. Her ability to communicate with the school and health professionals is limited because of her inability to speak English. She believes that her care as a mother is important for her daughter, and her goal is to see her daughter

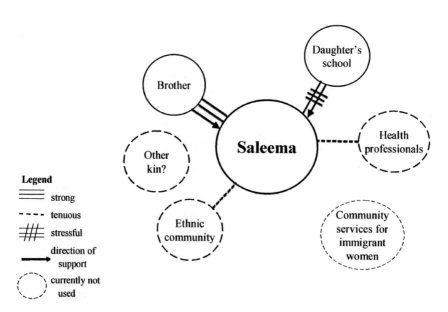

Figure 8.5. Ecomap of supportive and nonsupportive interactions for Saleema.

improve. Saleema's ecomap illustrates a lack of support, with heavy reliance on her brother, who was her sponsor for immigration. There is stress in her relationship with her daughter's school. A professional working with Saleema may want to explore in more detail her process and considerations in seeking support. Are there others who have assisted her in the past or with whom she has exchanged assistance? What is her relationship with her brother, and what considerations does she think about in seeking more help from him? When she had difficulty understanding the teachers at the school, how did she manage? How was she able to participate in the developmental assessment of her daughter? In her case there may be potential for additional aid through others in her ethnic community, other kin, or perhaps her brother and his family. In particular, does she know any health professionals who speak her language and who might be able to help her identify and connect with services such as programs for immigrant women, including English language instruction? Her primary link to services currently is her child's school, which may offer additional support for families of which she is unaware. Taking a more "upstream" perspective, community health nurses, social workers, and outreach workers may choose to become active in health and social planning committees to develop ways to more effectively contact and support immigrant women in their community who need assistance. They might advocate for increased access to interpreters who speak Punjabi, or develop pamphlets on health and social services written in Punjabi for distribution to ethnic organizations, community centers, and health and social care professionals. They may also choose to advocate for improved access to English language instruction for immigrant women.

CONCLUSION

Our goal in this chapter was to provide an overview of caregivers' experience of support as generated from the findings of our research. A sensitizing framework of support in the context of family caregiving can assist clinicians to more readily recognize cues and patterns in the experience of social support over time. By identifying common factors influencing a caregiver's access to support, it may be possible for health professionals to generate options for exploration and to facilitate the caregiver's access to support with increased sensitivity. Ultimately, such knowledge must be integrated with other knowledge in formulating clinical judgments. Clinicians need to consider the fit of our suggestions in the context of their experience in practice, their relationship with the client, the context of their practice, and their clinical judgment.

REFERENCES

Barbour, R. S. (2000). The role of qualitative research in broadening the "evidence base" for clinical practice. *Journal of Evaluation and Clinical Practice, 6*(2), 155–163.

Berkman, L., Glass, T., Brissette, I., & Seeman, T. (2000). From social integration to health: Durkheim in the new millennium. *Social Science & Medicine, 51,* 843–857.

Eisner, M., & Wright, M. (1986) A feminist approach to general practice. In C. Webb (Ed.), *Feminist practice in women's health care* (pp. 113–145) New York: Wiley.

Hooyman, N. R., & Gonyea, J. G. (1999) A feminist model of family care: Practice and policy directions. *Journal of Women & Aging, 11*(2), 149–169.

Kearney, M. H. (2001). Levels and applications of qualitative research evidence. *Research in Nursing & Health, 24,* 145–153.

Legault, A., & Ducharme, F. (2009). Advocating for a parent with dementia in a long-term care facility. *Journal of Family Nursing, 15,* 198–219.

Morse, J. M., Hutchinson, S. A., & Penrod, J. (1998). From theory to practice: The development of assessment guides from qualitatively derived theory. *Qualitative Health Research, 8,* 329–340.

Rafaeli, E., & Gleason, M. E. J. (2009). Skilled support within intimate relationships. *Journal of Family Theory & Review, 1,* 20–37.

Sandelowski, M. (1997). "To be of use": Enhancing utility of qualitative research. *Nursing Outlook, 45*(3), 125–132.

———. (2004). Using qualitative research. *Qualitative Health Research, 14*(10), 1366–1386.

Wright, L. M., & Leahy, M. (2005). *Nurses and families: A guide to family assessment and intervention* (4th ed.). Philadelphia: F. A. Davis.

Methodological Approaches: Lessons Learned

Nurses and other health professionals work with vulnerable populations, including family caregivers. It is important in research with populations such as family caregivers to recognize their vulnerability and to provide them with the supportive conditions to choose what they will share in their own words and in the setting of their choice. In this section of the book, we discuss methodological lessons learned in our research program with family caregivers that may be useful for researchers in practice settings. We describe our use of ecomaps and genograms to portray social networks (Chapter 9), our use of a card sort technique with think aloud interviews to generate data in interviews and focus groups (Chapter 10), and the approaches we used to facilitate the participation of immigrant women in research (Chapter 11).

We first present a discussion of the use of genograms and ecomaps as research tools. Although these instruments were developed for practice, we have found them to be useful in research. We illustrate their use with examples from a study of men caring for a relative with dementia. Although data from the study used as an illustration of ecomaps and genograms in Chapter 9 were not included in our presentation in previous chapters,[1] our use of these tools in previous studies was similar. In our experience, these tools were a valuable catalyst for generating additional information and reflection from participants and a useful vehicle for documenting key information about sources of support. We argue that there is potential for application of these tools with diverse research methods, family caregiving situations, and participants. An additional query is whether they also have unutilized potential as a catalyst in generating detailed information about family caregiving situations that may be useful in practice.

Our use of the card sort exercise (Chapter 10) was guided by our interest in developing a typology of nonsupportive interactions. Initially we conducted in-depth interviews with caregivers. From those interviews, we selected key quotations that reflected recurring themes and prepared a list of statements describing supportive and nonsupportive interactions. The statements were incorporated into an exercise with research participants in which they talked aloud to a researcher about their decisions while sorting cards into piles representing their perception of what was a supportive or nonsupportive. We learned the value of using phrases close to the participants' own words, recognized that participants interpreted the same statements in different ways, and found that multiple rehearsals of the exercise by the researchers were invaluable preparation. Although we do not describe it in the article that follows, we also effectively used card sort statements as a basis for discussion in focus groups with caregivers and professionals at the end of a study. We raise the question of whether a similar approach could be developed for application in a support group program.

In the final chapter in this section, we discuss some of the issues we addressed in our study of South Asian immigrant women. Encouraging members of vulnerable groups to participate in research in a way that values their contribution and empowers them is a challenge for all researchers. As a research team, we faced this issue particularly when working with immigrant women, who were vulnerable, not only as family caregivers but also by their minority status in the larger society as newcomers who often had limited economic resources and facility in the English language. The approaches we used are often considered specific to populations with language and or cultural diversity, but they can be helpful with other vulnerable populations. The approaches we chose were intended to address power differentials and included employment of multilingual interviewers from the participants' communities, the incorporation of an advisory committee, extensive advance piloting of interview guides, and support for participants' expenses.

NOTE

1. A report of the study used for the illustration of our use of ecomaps and genograms can be found in: Neufeld, A. & Kushner, K. (2009). Men family caregivers' experience of nonsupportive interactions: Context and expectations. *Journal of Family Nursing 15*(2), 171–197.

9

Data Generation: Interactive Use of Genograms and Ecomaps

Family caregiving research contributes to a body of knowledge that informs clinical practice with families across the life span. This research also generates innovative research methods to examine the dynamics of family caregiving, including the experience of supportive and nonsupportive interactions (which include absence of expected support). The use of genograms and ecomaps (see Figures 9.1 and 9.2) is a valuable research strategy to provide a "visual means of facilitating discussions around the structure and strengths of networks" (Ray & Street, 2005, p. 545), although their original and predominant application is in family therapy and clinical family nursing. We argue for their increased utilization as a data generation method based on our experience of their contribution in a study of male family caregivers' experiences of supportive and nonsupportive interactions.

The purpose of this chapter is to consider the use of genograms and ecomaps as heuristic tools in family caregiving research through examples of their use in our family caregiving research. These tools are graphic portrayals of family structure (genogram) and social relationships (ecomap; Wright & Leahey, 2005). In our research with family caregivers, these paper-and-pencil activities depicted the caregivers' descriptions of their family structure and social networks, including supportive and nonsupportive relationships that incorporated health-related resources. Our goal is to address the methodological use of genograms and ecomaps in research, not to report study findings.

Date: *Composite*
Code: *Composite*

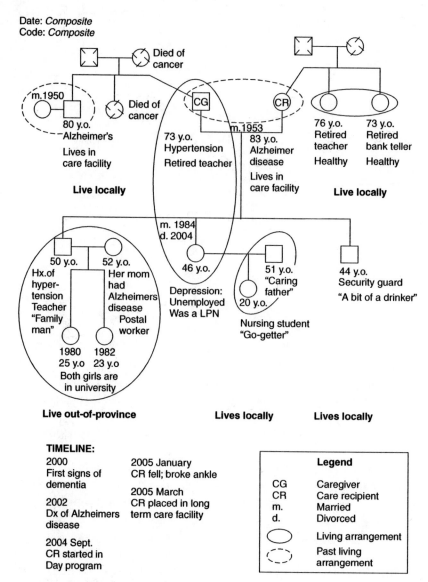

Figure 9.1. Example of a genogram.

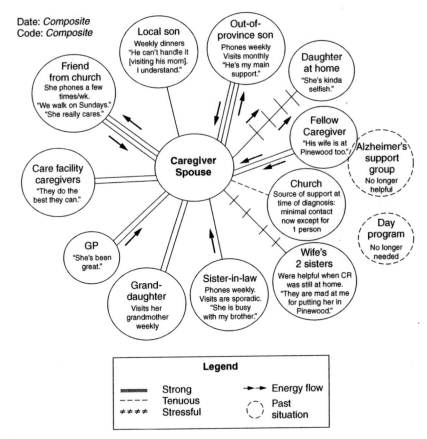

Figure 9.2. Example of an ecomap.

The interactive use of genograms and ecomaps in our research involved constructing and analyzing these diagrams concurrently and comparatively in conjunction with qualitative research interviews. The outcomes of this process included development of a rich contextual foundation for social support network research, a relational posture between the researcher and participant, and generation of useful questions during the data generation and analysis phases of research. Our concurrent and comparative use of genograms and ecomaps enabled us to identify new information such as the presence of shadow networks with potential for caregiver support within the participant's network of kin, friends, and professionals. For the purpose of this chapter, we will use examples from our current ethnographic study of perceptions of supportive and nonsupportive interactions of men caring for a spouse or parent with dementia. We have used genograms and ecomaps in other studies of perceptions of supportive and nonsupportive interactions of women and men in diverse family caregiving situations (Neufeld & Harrison, 1995, 1998; Neufeld, Harrison, Hughes, & Stewart, 2007; Neufeld & Kushner, 2009) as well as in a study of parenting children with life-threatening heart disease (Rempel, 2005). Literature reflecting the use of genograms and ecomaps in research is limited.

BACKGROUND

Genograms and ecomaps are used extensively in clinical practice with families, less often in the preparation of clinicians, and rarely in research. Especially useful from a systems perspective, genograms help the clinician to diagram the members of a family in relation to each other, often including three generations, with a view to detecting repeated patterns (McGoldrick, Gerson, & Shellenberger, 1999). Genograms and ecomaps have appeared in the family nursing literature since the introduction of the Calgary Family Assessment Model in 1984 (Wright & Leahey, 1984). Although genograms have come to be used worldwide in diverse family situations, critique of the device as positivistic (Milewski-Hertlein, 2001) and based on traditional views of the family has led to further development of the tool to reflect diversity related to culture, gender, sexuality, and spirituality. For example, conventional genogram format has been revised to reflect different religious affiliations (Frame, 2000); diverse cultures (Watts-Jones, 1997); cultural variables of ethnicity, gender, immigration, social class, and spirituality (Thomas, 1998); and alternative family situations (Milewski-Hertlein, 2001).

The information garnered from ecomaps concerns the social networks of an individual or family and the nature of the bonds within their networks (Hartman, 1995). For assessment and intervention purposes, awareness of the extent and nature of one's social network is helpful for the clinician and the client. For example, Hodge (2000) developed spiritual ecomaps to assess the role that spirituality plays in one's life and to provide information potentially useful in clinical practice with families. Although clinicians often use genograms and ecomaps in family therapy, implying a longer term and focused family-clinician relationship, Wright and Leahey have proposed the 15-minute family interview that includes completing a genogram and ecomap with the individual client in acute care settings (Wright & Leahey, 1999, 2005). Utility of this innovative clinical application is becoming evident in the literature (Holtslander, 2005).

In education programs, clinicians learn to use genograms and ecomaps in their clinical work with families. They also gain self-knowledge through intentional personal use of these tools to promote both self-awareness and sensitivity. For example, students construct ethical genograms and spiritual and cultural genograms and ecomaps to enhance understanding of their own backgrounds and to sensitize them to potential influences on their practice with families (Halevy, 1998; Keiley et al., 2002; Peluso, 2006).

There is emerging, although scant, evidence in the literature of genogram and ecomap use in research. Our search of health science literature published in English identified four studies. In three of the four studies, only one of the tools was used, either the genogram or the ecomap. Watts and Shrader (1998) utilized genograms to explore the presence of violence against women in Zimbabwe and Latin America. These researchers offered genograms as a research interview tool to document patterns of decision making, conflict, and vulnerability within families. Helling and Stovers (2005) suggested that genograms are useful in studies where family researchers are interviewing multiple family members. In their research with families transferring ranches from one generation to another, Helling and Stovers interviewed three to eight family members from each family. Participants completed a genogram prior to the interview. The genogram provided a basis for formulating key interview questions and was helpful in ensuring that the researchers considered all family members for an interview. Helling and Stovers recommended that researchers use the genograms early in the data generation phase and that they keep them simple.

Ray and Street (2005) employed ecomaps in their study of caregivers of people living with motor neuron disease. The researchers were particularly interested in mapping supportive networks of "carers" to identify actual and potential sources of nurture. Ray co-constructed the ecomap with the participant during the first interview and presented the ecomap at the second and third interviews to discuss and map changes since the previous interview. This study highlighted the collaborative potential of the mapping exercise and the utility of the ecomap tool in documenting changes in a caregiver's support network over time. We found one study in which the researcher employed genograms and ecomaps concurrently. Yanicki (2005) argued for the use of "clinical tools" in research with disadvantaged families whose vocabulary was limited and who tended to be more concrete in their thinking. She proposed that the genogram and ecomap exercises would enhance the low-income single mothers' descriptions of their family support from home visitation.

UTILITY OF GENOGRAMS AND ECOMAPS IN OUR CURRENT RESEARCH

The concurrent and interactive use of genograms and ecomaps to enhance the qualitative data generated in semistructured interviews in our family caregiving research had several advantages. The process of constructing the genogram and ecomap and the completed depictions provided a rich context for understanding the social networks of the caregivers who participated in our research. The collaborative diagramming between the researcher and participant facilitated a relational process that led to in-depth conversation and further disclosure of participants' experiences of supportive and nonsupportive interactions. Use of these tools supported the ongoing and iterative question-posing integral to qualitative data generation and analysis. The process of genogram and ecomap construction generated additional interview questions. Concurrent and comparative analyses of the completed genograms and ecomaps stimulated further questions useful in ongoing analysis of the interview data. Moreover, comparing the genograms and ecomaps during analysis uncovered findings that would not have been apparent had we only used one tool or used both but analyzed them separately. Each of these advantages will be discussed in depth, drawing on illustrations from our research experience.

Rich Contextual Foundation

The interviewer drafted a genogram and ecomap following the first interview and presented them both to the participant during a second interview for confirmation, refinement, and further development. Both the process of creating participant genograms and ecomaps based on data from the first interview and the subsequent data generated provided a rich context for understanding the social support network of each male caregiver and contributed new perspectives useful in data analysis.

We enhanced our understanding of the contextual influences on men's capacity for caregiving by incorporating in the genogram selected individual and family data beyond the traditional diagramming of each person's biological and legal place in the family, birth and marriage dates, and health conditions of various family members. Our expanded geno-gram data can be characterized by McGoldrick and colleagues' (1999) designation of demographic information, functional information (i.e., objective data on the medical, emotional, and behavioral functioning of different family members), and critical family events. Specifically, we incorporated demographic information from the first interview regarding age, birth and death dates, geographical location, living arrangements, occupation, and education level. We selected these key demographic characteristics to augment our understanding of the caregiver's context in preparation for the second interview and to facilitate the participant's reflection on social support experiences during the course of the second interview. The pictorial nature of the enhanced genograms prompted the men to further describe their caregiving context. For example, the visual presence of Alzheimer's disease in other family members and doc-umentation of their care situation (e.g., in care facility or being cared for at home) led participants to describe the influence of those data on their current caregiving situation.

Information about how individuals functioned within the family included the participant's positive or negative comments on emotional or behavioral patterns (e.g., "caring father") as well as health status where relevant. We inserted these comments near the symbols that rep-resented the corresponding family member. We incorporated critical family events into the genogram, often as a note off to the side. Critical events reflected relational losses and gains in the family through birth, death, separation, divorce, illness, and conflict. On the genogram, we also constructed a timeline of critical events related to the care recipi-ent's illness (see Figure 9.1).

The augmented genogram data alerted us to geographic, employ-ment, and health issues that may have influenced potential family mem-bers' ability to provide help with caregiving as well as changes in the living situation of the caregiver and care recipient. Our focus on supportive and nonsupportive interactions determined what additional genogram information we pursued. This information proved useful in enriching our understanding of the caregiving context, including the potential for support mobilization or lack thereof. For example, changes in living arrangements were common in our sample of male family caregivers, and we intentionally captured these data by encircling the members of a household with a solid circle and previous household configurations with a broken line circle. In this way, we gained a pictorial depiction of house-hold changes that stimulated interview conversation about experiences of supportive and nonsupportive interactions based on living arrangements. Regarding employment details, one participant, who was a retired teacher, proudly talked about his three daughters who were all teachers, one of whom recently had retired. From a researcher's perspective, this relevant genogram data led to conversation during the ecomap exercise about factors related to the support he received from his daughters that included and went beyond their employment as teachers.

Ecomap data enhanced our understanding of the caregiving context by identifying key sources of support, including connections with kin, friends, affiliations or club memberships, employers, and professionals (see Figure 9.2). Each circle placed on the ecomap represented a relationship that influenced the caregiver's experience of caregiving. We depicted the nature of the relationship, including the dimensions of energy flow (i.e., reciprocal or one-way exchanges), intensity, and stress. We identified tenuous relationships on the ecomap as well as support sources that were no longer helpful or relevant. We depicted these by broken lines. We added comments regarding frequency of contacts, indicating, for example, daily phone calls in comparison to monthly visits. Caregivers' comments pertaining to personality traits of others that seemed linked to their capacity to provide support were included on the ecomap more often than on the genogram, but this documentation decision was arbitrary at times.

Key findings from our ecomap data related to the changing support networks of male family caregivers of a relative with dementia. Whereas relationships with family members remained relatively stable, either as sources of supportive or nonsupportive interactions, there were changes over time in friends and professionals as support sources. Ecomap data, namely broken line circles, clearly depicted the friends who had fallen away since the care recipient's onset of dementia, an evident pattern among the study participants. Participants identified some friends as a continuing source of support as well as a new network of friends that developed for some of the men. Often these friendships arose from the support sources that the caregiver accessed because of the care recipient's illness. For example, many participants made acquaintances through advocacy and support groups, and in some cases meaningful and enduring friendships formed. Another source of new friendships was through the formal caregiving network. One caregiver gained a special friendship with a person who worked at the facility where he had first placed his wife with advanced Alzheimer's disease. We depicted these newly acquired supports by a "circle out of a circle" that showed that the friendship arose from a formal source of support. Several men in the study had participated in support groups in the early stages of their relative's dementia. Although the support group was no longer a key source of support, some of the men remained in contact with a friend that they had made during their time in the support group. In this situation, the solid circle coming out of the broken-line circle showed the ongoing friendship that had arisen from a past source of support.

The genogram and ecomap data provided a rich context for analysis of participants' perceptions of supportive and nonsupportive interactions as well as a means of comparing the networks of subgroups of caregivers and of exploring patterns of support over time. For example, when comparing the networks of sons and spouses, we noted a pattern of fewer supports for son caregivers as compared to male spousal caregivers. Sons tended not to involve themselves in support groups and did not identify fellow caregivers as sources of support in the same way as spouses did.

Participant—Researcher Relationship

Both the collaborative nature of genogram and ecomap data generation and the appeal that the tools had for the participants contributed to rapport and exchange between the participant and the interviewer. This development, in turn, facilitated participants' freedom of communication and rich descriptions of their experiences of supportive and nonsupportive interactions as caregivers.

The relational process of jointly diagramming the family structure and support network stimulated reflection for the interviewer and participant that led to conversation about the participant's family and descriptions of experiences of supportive and nonsupportive interactions. The atmosphere of equality promoted by the joint efforts of the interviewer and participant in creating the genograms and ecomaps facilitated rapport. Sometimes this rapport led to disclosure of sensitive family information, often not easily shared with a stranger (i.e., the interviewer). For example, one participant, in the context of drawing the genogram, disclosed that his wife had not been able to handle being a mother and so other family members had raised their two sons. He pointed these family members out on the genogram as he related this sensitive information. During the process of genogram and ecomap construction, some men also identified a significant relationship with another woman that had arisen during the course of their spouse's illness. It seemed important to the men that they reveal the significant support they received from this new woman in their life, and the ecomap exercise presented them with a nonthreatening opportunity to share this sensitive information. Giving the woman a place on the eco-map was a way of validating the relationship, and we respected the sensitive nature of this revelation in the conversation that ensued.

The participants' positive responses to the genogram and ecomap also played a role in stimulating self-reflection about their family history and context in relation to their current caregiving role. Rather than representing imposed research tools requiring completion, the genogram and ecomap captured the interest of participants and served as a catalyst for conversation. Participants remarked positively about what it was like to see their family members and support network mapped before them, and they were keen to provide detailed structural and network information. Some participants retrieved photographs of family members to show the interviewer. In one such situation, the picture showed only three grown children, rather than the four indicated on the genogram. After naming each child in the picture, the man told the story of one daughter's sudden death. An 89-year-old participant had a piece of folk art that included all of the birthdates of his children and grandchildren, and he brought the arrangement of decorated wooden hearts to the interview table to refer to as he provided detailed genogram information.

One man, highly engaged with the diagrams, removed them from the interviewer's hand, set them in front of himself and began making his own entries, documenting where his out-of-town siblings lived. He referred to the genogram and ecomap throughout the interview and concluded that the ecomap would be a helpful tool for him to reflect on his support network periodically as he cared for his wife with Alzheimer's disease.

Concurrent and Comparative Use

A further advantage of using genograms and ecomaps interactively in our research was that their concurrent and comparative use uncovered data that may not have been apparent had we not used the tools, used only one, or used them separately from each other. During the course of the interview, the interviewer had the opportunity to raise questions about the genogram and ecomap. For example, the interviewer could ask about interactions with particular family members who were on the genogram but not on the ecomap. When a caregiver's support network consisted primarily of professional caregivers rather than family members, the interviewer could ask a question such as, "What is it like to have so many professionals in your life?" or "What is it like for you to only see your children on special occasions?"

The main finding that arose from our concurrent and comparative genogram and ecomap use was the identification of unrealized potential in the participants' support networks that we came to identify as their "shadow" network. For example, one caregiver explained that the reason his daughter, who lived "down the street," was not included on the ecomap was her extensive family and employment responsibilities. He also commented that he did not expect her to help him with his caregiving, so this relationship was not a source of stress or disappointment for him. His relationship with his daughter was not a source of either support or nonsupport. In both the kin and professional realm, there was opportunity to ask participants to reflect on potential sources of support that apparently they had not fully realized. The circumstances of and possible reasons for this could then be explored. This exploration helped us identify the conditions that contributed to the experience of supportive and nonsupportive interactions for male caregivers in this study.

The genogram and ecomap data also revealed changes in the support network over time. The genograms and ecomaps were initially constructed using data from the first interview and then updated and revised when taken back to the participants in the second interview. Participants also identified sources of support that were helpful early in their caregiving experience but were no longer helpful at the time of the interview. For example, most men identified support groups for caregivers of relatives with Alzheimer's disease as less helpful as their caregiving experience progressed and their focus shifted from securing information about the disease to securing resources to sustain caregiving.

A key aspect of data analysis was to examine each participant's genogram and ecomap to answer the following questions: Which genogram members did not appear on the ecomap? and What genogram information available (e.g., geography, illness, death, and family dynamics) helped to explain the presence or absence of support? This analysis revealed patterns of supportive and nonsupportive interaction that we then further explored in the analysis of interview data.

CASE ILLUSTRATION

To illustrate our use of these tools, we present a composite case illustration derived from data in a study of male caregivers (Neufeld & Kushner, 2009), of a 73-year-old retired schoolteacher whose spouse received a diagnosis of Alzheimer's disease 4 years prior to the study (see Figures 9.1 and 9.2). At the time of our first interview, this man was caring for his wife in their family home. At the second interview, 6 months later, she had been in a care facility for 4 months. Through the process of drawing the genogram, the interviewer noted that a number of family members lived locally, including a son and daughter, and that living arrangements for the caregiver had changed recently. Because his wife was no longer living at home with him, he now shared his home with his recently divorced daughter. The caregiver indicated that the two younger sisters of his wife lived together and were healthy. The caregiver's brother was in the late stages of Alzheimer's disease and lived in a care facility. Based on the genogram alone, one might assume a potential network of support within the caregiver's family, including his daughter who was living with him, his son, and his sisters-in-law. Through the process of drawing the ecomap, it became clear, however, that this man's main support was his son who lived in another province. The son and daughter who lived locally were emotionally unavailable due to their own family, employment, and health issues, and were unable to offer practical support to assist their father in caregiving. The caregiver expressed gratitude that his local son initiated a weekly dinner out, "although I always pay" was his added comment. During the ecomapping exercise, it also became evident that the caregiver's two sisters-in-law had been supportive before their sister's placement in a care facility. The caregiver stated that the sisters were angry with him for placing his wife in a care facility and no longer initiated contact with him but visited their sister regularly.

Our case illustration also draws attention to the changes that occur within the support networks of caregivers. The Alzheimer's support group, as depicted by a lighter circle, is no longer helpful for the caregiver, but he gained a friend from this past source of support that we have depicted as "a circle out of a circle." The church remains as a source of possible support, although the broken line of connection indicates the tenuousness of the relationship, as he no longer attends services regularly.

REFLECTIONS AND IMPLICATIONS FOR FURTHER RESEARCH

Similar to the diverse applications of genograms and ecomaps in clinical practice and in the education of clinicians, we propose that there is potential for diverse application in research. For example, researchers can use genograms and ecomaps with different methodological approaches and methods, different caregiving situations, and diverse research participants.

Potential Application in Diverse Methodological Approaches and Methods

Genograms and ecomaps are adaptable research tools that have utility in diverse qualitative study designs in family nursing research. Use of these tools, for example, could elicit stories such as those generated in narrative inquiry. Participants' descriptions of changes over time would elicit process data integral to grounded theory research. Opportunity to identify differences between participants' ecomaps in home and long-term care settings could yield data amenable to critical analysis. In our ethnographic study, data about support networks generated with an individual family member through the genogram and ecomap exercises provided rich contextual data. In a mixed-methods approach, we envision the potential utility of quantifying the ecomap data to detect trends in the data or to develop taxonomies of caregiving networks. Varied sampling, data generation, and data analysis methods also lend themselves to genogram and ecomap utilization, assuming that the practical and ethical implications receive due consideration.

Use of various sampling strategies, such as including multiple family members individually, conjointly, or as a family group, could present issues of confidentiality and serial documentation for our consideration. For example, if all family members contribute to the construction of one composite genogram in their individual interviews, confidentiality is a concern. Sharing the genogram or ecomap data with other family members requires participant permission or consent, even though one might consider the construction of a genogram, for example, as the gathering of factual, objective information. "Bare bones" genogram data pertaining to family composition including birth, marriage, and death dates appears straightforward. Even in this regard, however, different family members may have different knowledge or recall regarding birthdates and anniversaries, for example, and different sensitivities about other family members' "getting it right." Unless researchers specify in the research design the sharing of data generated individually from multiple family members, the data collected in the context of an individual research interview are confidential.

Researchers can address this issue of confidentiality through an evolving or emergent research design whereby they negotiate with family members to reach agreement about sharing genogram and/or ecomap data with other family members either separately or together in a family interview. The researcher is asking the participants to consider sharing the genogram and/or ecomap data only, not all interview data. Reaching consensus among multiple family members regarding the family's genogram and collective family or household ecomap is a source of family-level interactional data in addition to the outcomes of the paper-and-pencil exercises.

Implications for documentation include whether and how to record the contributions of each family member on a composite genogram or ecomap. We propose using one color of pen or pencil with the first family member and different colors with subsequent family members to track who contributed which data. Depending on the configuration of various family members, another method may be that all data provided by sons, for example, be one particular color and all data from spouses another color.

Depending on the purpose of the research and specific research questions, the researcher could generate genogram and ecomap data from individual family members and then compare findings in the context of a family interview or, alternatively, as an analytic process without the family's input. Circular questions regarding genogram or ecomap entries in the context of a research interview can yield additional relational data for analysis. For example, the interviewer could ask a woman what it is like for her to see that her husband did not include her on his ecomap when she included him on her ecomap. Both the nature and content of her response yields data for analysis.

Potential for Application in Diverse Family Caregiving Situations

The adaptable nature of genograms and ecomaps in research also ensures their utility in research about diverse family caregiving situations. In our study, Alzheimer's disease or other dementias represented a chronic and progressive disease, and data generation occurred over time to capture the changes in supportive and nonsupportive caregiving interactions as the disease progressed. We portrayed these changes on the genogram and ecomap. One could also capture changes in social networks related to critical or episodic illnesses that resolve and/or change related to developmental changes in families. When constructing the genograms and ecomaps prospectively during multiple interviews, we suggest documenting "Time 1" data in one color of pencil or pen and "Time 2" data in another color as we did in an earlier study (Neufeld & Harrison, 1995).

In our ongoing research programs, we continue to employ genograms and ecomaps as data generation tools and anticipate their continued utility in studies of diverse caregiving situations. For example, in family caregiving research related to transitions for parents when healthy babies are born and when babies are born with life-threatening conditions, use of genograms and ecomaps can facilitate generation of information about intergenerational support. As we follow families longitudinally, the ecomaps of individual family members demonstrate how caregiving realities change through normal developmental stages and illness-related events. Use of genograms and ecomaps as research tools may contribute to generation of data that facilitate understanding of family health dynamics.

Potential Application to Diverse Research Participants

The user appeal of the genogram and ecomap as research tools means that they are potentially adaptable to participants of different age, gender, generation, cognition, and command of the English language. Our study included several immigrants and frail older participants. The tools worked well for them. The pictorial nature of the tools contributes to their effective use with people whose first language is not English or with those whose comprehension of abstract questions is limited. This broad user appeal holds particular potential for intergenerational support research.

For example, in our ongoing research about transition to parenthood and intergenerational support, we employ genograms and ecomaps with parents and grandparents. In research with parents and adolescents to assess readiness for transitioning youth from specialized pediatric care settings to adult care settings, we can depict gains and losses in the social networks of youth and their families through serial genograms and ecomaps in research interviews with adult parents and their adolescents.

We are curious about potential for application of these tools with children and predict that both tools would have appeal for this age group as well. Connolly (2005) has proposed the use of self-created genograms in which she asks students and clients to draw their family. She has found that this nontraditional creative approach to diagramming one's family ensures that nontraditional family structure is captured and sensitive issues are disclosed that can be discussed through further conversations. This may have application for children.

On the basis of our experience, we believe that genograms and eco-maps are especially effective in furthering conversation with men, whatever their age or generation. In our caregiving research with women, we found that they typically were forthcoming regarding sensitive relational issues, such as relational strain with other family members. In comparison, men were not as forthcoming, but the interactive use of genograms and ecomaps facilitated more in-depth discussion. Our ongoing research with adolescents, parents, and grandparents provides opportunity for us to analyze for gender differences in response to the use of genograms and ecomaps in research.

CONCLUSION

We see the potential for genuine collaboration in the interactive co-construction of genograms and ecomaps with family caregivers who are willing to share their experiences for the purposes of research and knowledge development. We contend that much of the power of genograms and ecomaps in family caregiving research exists in the relational stance that this collaborative activity facilitates. In our experience, the concurrent and comparative use of genograms and ecomaps in family caregiving research was effective. It enhanced our understanding of social networks as a context for caregiving, and promoted and uncovered findings that may not have become evident with the use of the tools singly or separately.

NOTE

Originally published in Rempel, G., Neufeld, A., & Kushner, K. E. (2007). Interactive use of genograms and ecomaps in family caregiving research. *Journal of Family Nursing, 13*(4), 403–419.

REFERENCES

Connolly, C. M. (2005). Discovering "family" creatively: The self-created genogram. *Journal of Creativity in Mental Health, 1*(1), 81–105.

Frame, M. W. (2000). The spiritual genogram in family therapy. *Journal of Marital & Family Therapy, 26*(2), 211–216.

Halevy, J. (1998). A genogram with an attitude. *Journal of Marital & Family Therapy, 24*(2), 233–242.

Hartman, A. (1995). Diagrammatic assessment of family relationships. *Families in Society: The Journal of Contemporary Human Services, 76*(2), 111–122.

Helling, M. K., & Stovers, R. G. (2005). Genogram as a research tool. *Great Plains Sociologist, 17*(1), 78–85.

Hodge, D. R. (2000). Spiritual ecomaps: A new diagrammatic tool for assessing marital and family spirituality. *Journal of Marital & Family Therapy, 26*(2), 217–228.

Holtslander, L. (2005). Clinical application of the 15-minute family interview: Addressing the needs of postpartum families. *Journal of Family Nursing, 11*(1), 5–18.

Keiley, M. K., Dolbin, M., Hill, J., Karuppaswamy, N., Liu, T., Natrajan, R., et al. (2002). The cultural genogram: Experiences from within a marriage and family therapy training program. *Journal of Marital & Family Therapy, 28*(2), 165–178.

McGoldrick, M., Gerson, R., & Shellenberger, S. (1999). *Genograms: Assessment and Intervention* (2nd ed.). New York: W. W. Norton.

Milewski-Hertlein, K. (2001). The use of a socially constructed genogram in clinical practice. *The American Journal of Family Therapy, 29*, 23–38.

Neufeld, A., & Harrison, M. J. (1995). Reciprocity and social support in caregivers' relationships: Variations and consequences. *Qualitative Health Research, 5*, 349–366.

———. (1998). Men as caregivers: Reciprocal relationships or obligation? *Journal of Advanced Nursing, 28*(5), 959–968.

Neufeld, A., Harrison, M. J., Hughes, K., & Stewart, M. (2007). Nonsupportive interactions in the experience of women family caregivers. *Health and Social Care in the Community, 15*(6), 530–541.

Neufeld, A., & Kushner, K. E. (2009). Men family caregivers' experience of nonsupportive interactions: Context and expectations. *Journal of Family Nursing, 15*(2), 171–191.

Peluso, P. R. (2006). Expanding the use of the ethical genogram: Incorporating the ethical principles to help clarify counselors' ethical decision-making styles. *The Family Journal: Counseling and Therapy for Couples and Families, 14*(2), 158–163.

Ray, R. A., & Street, A. F. (2005). Ecomapping: An innovative research tool for nurses. *Journal of Advanced Nursing, 50*(5), 545–552.

Rempel, G. R. (2005). *Parenting a child with HLHS whose treatment includes the Norwood surgical approach.* Unpublished doctoral dissertation, University of Alberta, Edmonton.

Thomas, A. J. (1998). Understanding culture and worldview in family systems: Use of the multicultural genogram. *The Family Journal: Counseling and Therapy for Couples and Families, 6*(1), 24–32.

Watts-Jones, D. (1997). Toward an African American genogram. *Family Process, 36*(4), 375–383.

Watts, C., & Shrader, E. (1998). The genogram: A new research tool to document patterns of decision-making, conflict and vulnerability within households. *Health Policy & Planning, 13*(4), 459–464.

Wright, L. M., & Leahey, M. (1984). *Nurses and families: A guide to family assessment and intervention.* Philadelphia: F. A. Davis.

———. (1999). Maximizing time, minimizing suffering: The 15-minute (or less) family interview. *Journal of Family Nursing, 5,* 259–274.

———. (2005). *Nurses and families: A guide to family assessment and intervention* (4th ed.). Philadelphia: F. A. Davis.

Yanicki, S. (2005). Social support and family assets. *Canadian Journal of Public Health, 96,* 46–49.

10

Using a Card Sort Technique in Data Generation

We found the use of a card sort data generation technique effective in both individual interviews and focus groups. We report in this chapter on our use of a card sort technique in our ethnographic study of women's appraisal of nonsupport experienced in the context of diverse family caregiving situations. The purpose of the card sort was to enable us to move from concrete examples to more abstract views of support and nonsupport that would facilitate development of a classification and description of types of nonsupport that women caregivers experience. The perspective of symbolic interaction (Prus, 1996) informed the approach in this study as we considered individuals' perceptions and actions within the context of social settings. As we prepared to initiate the card sort procedure, we found that although the use of card sorts is addressed in the research literature, practical information to guide the development and implementation of the procedure was limited. The purpose of this chapter is to share our reflections on the practical challenges encountered in using a card sort and the strategies we developed.

BACKGROUND

The card sort has been used as a qualitative data collection technique in many social science and health disciplines (Ryan & Bernard, 2000; Morse & Field, 1995). Sometimes called a pile sort, a card sort is a research data collection technique that enables researchers to gain information about the conceptual dimensions research participants use to appraise their social experience (Nastasi & Berg, 1999; Spradley, 1979). In ethnoscience, researchers have used the card sort to facilitate the construction of a taxonomy that portrays a hierarchical classification of the dimensions of a concept explored in the research (Miller & Crabtree, 1999; Morse & Field, 1995).

Use of card sorts has proliferated to encompass a wide variety of research and clinical applications. Different traditions have emphasized linguistic analysis of text, or analysis as a means of understanding experience (Ryan & Bernard, 2000). In a classic use of the card sort in an ethnographic study of "tramps," Spradley (1979) wrote terms on cards and asked informants to verify whether the cards included all the different types. Using another set of terms on cards, he asked participants to sort out those terms into piles that were more similar than different. Spradley argued that use of the card sort and structured questions made it easier for participants to take part in the research and enabled the researcher to explore the organization as well as the content of participants' knowledge. In addition, the card sort activity prevented the researcher from prematurely imposing analytic categories to organize data.

Some researchers have used this technique to address issues of conceptual similarity and ethnographic grounding (Bernard, 2000; Weller, 1998), as well as the categorical organization of concepts (Canter, Brown, & Groat, 1985). Others have employed card sorts to develop decision models (Beaver, Bogg, & Luker, 1999; Olson & Morse, 1996), to determine participants' priority goals (Lang & Carstensen, 2002), or to identify perceptions of the priority of client learning needs by clients, physicians, and nurses (Luniewski, Reigle, & White, 1999). The card sort technique has also been used to aid in the design of interventions (Nastasi & Berg, 1999). For example, researchers have used the procedure to determine health care consumers' preferred roles in treatment decision making (Davison & Degner, 1997). Because it is a concrete task, card sorts are also appropriate for use with children. Roos (1998) used words and phrases in a study of preadolescent children's classification of foods. Johnson and Griffith (1998) reported using card sort pictures instead of written statements in their research on recognition of different fish species. The research context in which the card sort procedure is used will influence decisions about the specific protocol for administration and the practical challenges to be addressed.

RESEARCH CONTEXT: STUDY OF NONSUPPORT AND FAMILY CAREGIVING

The focus of our ethnographic study was to identify types of nonsupport that women in diverse family caregiving situations experienced. In the context of this research, we chose diverse situations to reflect variations in psychosocial characteristics and family caregiving demands associated with the care recipient's health condition. Characteristics of the care recipient's health condition that might be influential for support and nonsupport during caregiving include immediate or gradual onset, continuous or episodic occurrence, visible or invisible limitations, stigmatizing or nonstigmatizing features, and potential for loss of the relationship with the care recipient (Rolland, 1990, 1993, 1994). The specific purpose of the card sort activity was to elicit detailed information to facilitate development of a classification and description of types of nonsupport that women caregivers experienced.

The sample of women family caregivers in the larger study ($n = 59$) included women caring for infants born prematurely (immediate onset; $n = 15$), for children with asthma (episodic) or diabetes (continuous occurrence; $n = 14$), or for adult relatives with cancer (slow to develop, potential for loss; $n = 15$) or dementia (stigmatizing, invisible; $n = 15$). All women in the study were English speaking, some ($n = 6$) had less than grade 12 education, most had a partner ($n = 49$), and their annual family income ranged from less than CDN\$20,000 to more than \$80,000. More than half of the women ($n = 33$) participated in more than one data collection activity during the three years of data collection. Before the card sort interviews, sources of data included in-depth semistructured interviews, participant observation field notes, and caregiver diaries. Of the 59 women, 17 were included in the card sort phase of the study. Of these 17 women, 9 were participants in earlier phases of the study and were selected for the card sort on the basis of variation in caregiving situation. We included 8 new participants to provide information about the relevance of the items for other women in similar caregiving situations. Women newly recruited at the time of the card sort were demographically similar to the women who had taken part in earlier phases of the research.

The local institutional ethics review board approved the study. All participants signed a consent form prior to participation in the study and were advised that their participation was voluntary and that they were free to withdraw at any time.

PRACTICAL ISSUES AND STRATEGIES IN USING A CARD SORT FOR DATA COLLECTION

We faced several challenges in formulating the card sort statements and determining an effective protocol to address the issues that women faced in completing the exercise. In formulating appropriate statements, we experienced a tension between creating statements that were a meaningful reflection of the study data and statements that were manageable in the context of a structured card sort procedure. We also needed to address procedural, participant, and data collection challenges.

Procedural Issues

Meaningful Statements

We sought to develop meaningful statements that reflected the key themes previously identified from data analysis. We based the statements constructed for the card sort on an extensive database of prior interviews, diaries, and participant observation field notes. Because women from diverse caregiving situations would complete the card sort task, we needed to create statements that would be relevant to four different situations and could be meaningful without inclusion of detail about context. To achieve this goal, the first two authors reviewed the initial data in detail and generated matrix tables using the N6 (Nonnumerical Unstructured Data Indexing Searching and Theorizing) qualitative data analysis software to display the distribution of themes across the family caregiving situations. We then extracted from the data 274 quotations that reflected these key themes. We selected quotations portraying nonsupport and support or experiences that could be perceived as either support or nonsupport. We included statements describing support to clarify whether descriptions of nonsupport were a mirror image of support or conceptually different.

Criteria for further selection of quotations from this initial pool included attention to both similarity and diversity across groups, inclusion of as many themes as possible, and inclusion of family and friends as well as professionals as sources of support. Using these criteria, we reduced the number of selected quotations to 63. We formulated a statement that reflected the main idea in each quotation, trying to stay as close to the original quotation as possible. To construct statements that participants could understand without reference to the individual caregiving situation, we substituted general terms, such as "relative," "health care professional," or "agency" for specific references to "child," "husband," "nurse," "doctor," "hospital," or "long-term care unit." Two examples of final statements using generic terms are "The staff thought I was overprotective. They did not want to do as I asked" and "My relative looks OK. Others don't realize how ill she is and how much care she needs."

A Manageable Task

In the context of this study, we sought to engage participants in three card sort exercises, which each incorporated the same statements. In the first card sort, we asked women to sort statements into piles of cards that were similar in meaning and then to describe and label the piles they created. The participants could create as many piles as they wanted in this first sort, and the words or phrases they used to name the piles were entirely their own. This approach did not impose the researcher's perceptions or assumptions and has utility in gaining information about perceived similarities (Canter, Brown, & Groat, 1985). However, there is potential for participants to respond by creating either many piles that reflect detailed distinctions (splitters) or few piles reflecting only broad differences (lumpers; Borgatti, 1999; Weller & Romney, 1988). To address this lumper/splitter phenomenon, we used a constrained card sort that required a specified number of piles in each of the second and third card sort exercises. In the second sort, we asked participants to organize cards into three piles, indicating something that was helpful to them, something that was unhelpful, or something that was unclear. Participants placed cards in the unclear pile when they were unsure whether the statement represented something that was helpful or unhelpful, or when the statement did not immediately make sense for them in the context of their caregiving experience. In the final card sort, participants organized cards into two piles, indicating something that was helpful or unhelpful. To capture participants' initial reactions to the statements and the rationale for their choices, we asked them to describe their thinking out loud during the sort (Borgatti, 1999; Caulkins, 1998).

To ensure that the card sort task was manageable, the team of investigators participated in a feasibility pilot exercise of the card sort protocol in a workshop format. We role-played interviewer and participant roles using the initial 63 statements printed on 8.5 × 11" paper. On the basis of this experience, we reduced the total number of card statements to 30, to prevent participant fatigue and to ensure that the task was reasonable for the desired interview time of 1 to 1.5 hours. In addition, the statements were shortened and written at a grade 6 or lower reading level. Many statements were divided into two sentences. We also simplified the instructions and chose to use 4″ × 8″ cards of heavy paper to facilitate manipulation of the cards. In the second feasibility pilot, the interviewer conducted the card sort with a member of the project advisory committee who was also a family caregiver. This interview confirmed the utility of the statements constructed and the protocol developed. The 17 card sort interviews were then conducted and recorded on audiotape for transcription and analysis.

Challenges for Participants

Women caregivers faced several challenges as they engaged in the card sort exercise. For example, they often focused initially on their own experience, experienced test anxiety, or had an emotional response to card sort statements. We responded to these challenges by adjusting the card sort protocol.

Moving Beyond Their Experience

The women often shared details of their personal caregiving experience while engaged in the card sort task but found it difficult to move beyond their own experience to a more abstract level. In particular, the first card sort (in which choices were unconstrained) elicited women's stories. As they created, described out loud, and labeled piles of cards, they used their experience as the guide for their choices. Many developed a pile labeled "not my experience" and one labeled "my experience." In the second card sort (requesting helpful, unhelpful, or unclear piles), some women were initially unsure of how to respond to the card statements if all or part of a statement did not fit their experience. Although most women did make the shift to a more abstract level, others benefited from coaching to consider the statement in the context of family caregiving in general. One caregiver asked, "So do you mean helpful to me or helpful in general?" To this, the interviewer replied, "Thinking about your experience as a caregiver, does this statement reflect something that would be helpful or unhelpful for caregivers in general?" In reflecting on the card sort task, one woman said,

As the piles went on, it became more of an academic exercise. Like the last one [sort] was the easiest because I didn't have to decide whether I'd actually been through it or not, it was just generally, "Would that be something that was helpful or not?"

A strength of this card sort exercise was the combination of unconstrained and constrained sorts. Through the unconstrained sort, women identified key issues in caregiving based on their personal experience. Through the two constrained card sorts, women reflected on caregiving in general, as informed by their personal caregiving experiences.

Dealing with Test Anxiety

Test anxiety was another challenge participants faced. All of the women caregivers were conscientious in their approach to the card sort, carefully reviewed the written instructions, and asked questions for clarification. The card sort exercise felt like a "test" for some women, and they sought reassurance from the interviewer that their sorting decision was correct. Interviewer warmth and encouragement, and an unhurried interview pace helped to ease anxiety. One woman who was initially anxious but later relaxed said, "Your voice and the smile on your face . . . that makes all the difference."

The interviewer assured the women that "This is not a test." and "There are no right or wrong answers." Some women struggled with the context-free nature of the card statements. For example, the statement "They are right there when I need them." often elicited the question "Who does 'they' refer to?" The interviewer would respond with something like "It's up to you." or "You decide." Once the women overcame their anxiety, they enjoyed the card sort. One woman said it was like "playing cards."

Dealing with Emotional Responses

A third challenge for the women participants was the emotionally evocative nature of the card sort statements. As one woman said,

When you hear a certain song and it takes you back . . . certain cards that did the same thing; put you right back . . . in the hospital room . . . I wasn't expecting that.

One woman demonstrated her emotional response by laying some cards on the table with an emphatic motion. Emotions triggered by the statements included anger, hurt, disappointment, and sadness. Some women had to read all the statements through once to register some of their emotions before they could begin the card sorting exercise. For other women, reading the card statements aloud and talking out loud helped them to deal with their emotions:

> Well, you don't feel so pressured when you talk out loud . . . because it's going to explode, you know.

Reflecting on the evocative nature of the statements one caregiver commented,

> Emotions released can be like a freight train. . . . I will work very hard . . . so that those emotions and those experiences can settle back into their places.

The interviewer prepared participants at the beginning of the interview for the feelings they might experience. During the interview, she was sensitive to the need to respond in a caring manner when women cried, providing time to recover and talk about issues if needed. At the end of the interview, each woman was invited to describe her perceptions of the interview. In addition, the project coordinator maintained contact with participants by telephone, to give them an opportunity to comment on their participation and to inform them of available support resources.

Data Collection Challenges

Using a card sort exercise posed several challenges for data collection. These included achieving timely completion of the card sort task, eliciting the women's rationale for their card sort decisions, and accurate recording.

Timely Completion

To facilitate timely completion of the task, the interviewer telephoned the women in advance to arrange ample physical space to work with the cards (e.g., a dining room table) and uninterrupted time so the women could concentrate on the exercise. Many interviews were scheduled when the adult care recipient was away from the home at day care or the hospital, or when children were napping or at school. Because women wanted to share their stories, the interviewer sought to balance opportunity for relational storytelling with the task-oriented card sort. When women began to share their experiences during demographic data collection, the interviewer intentionally proceeded to the card sort as soon as possible, as there was ample time during the exercise for women to describe their experiences. This avoided repetition, kept the interview to the desired time frame, and helped to capture story elements that might otherwise have been lost.

Eliciting Rationale

To elicit the women caregivers' rationale for their card sort choices, as well as their initial reactions to the statements, we sought "think aloud" data from the participants (Borgatti, 1999; Caulkins, 1998). The interviewer encouraged the women to read the card statements aloud as they picked them up and to continue to think out loud, telling the interviewer the reasons they were placing the card in the selected pile. This strategy had several benefits. First, this think aloud data helped us to determine whether women who chose to place a card in a given pile did so for the same or different reasons as other women who put that card in the same pile. Second, this data provided useful information about the reasons that some women considered a statement helpful, whereas others viewed it as unhelpful, and assisted us in interpretation of results, including identification of the criteria they used in their appraisal. Third, the think aloud data allowed the interviewer to ensure that the woman placed the card in the intended pile. Occasionally, a woman would state her decision about a statement out loud but would inadvertently place the card in the opposite pile. The interviewer would then ask the woman what pile she intended, and the woman would correct her mistake. A limitation related to think aloud data was that participants were not always immediately able to explain the process that led to their sort choices. Some needed time to review and reconstruct what they had done before they could describe their rationale.

Accurate Recording

To establish an accurate record of the women's decisions, we created both audiotaped and written records of the card sort results. The interview transcription provided a record of the women's decisions and their rationale, and permitted verification of the accuracy of written records completed in the home. For ease of administration, we created three identical packages of cards and used one package for each card sort. We shuffled the cards prior to use so they would be presented in random order. We also placed card numbers on the back of each card to avoid distracting the participants or influencing their decisions. The interviewer recorded the results of each card sort on a record sheet. We retained the order in which cards were placed into piles in each package, for later use in checking the written record, and provided a new set for the next card sort.

REFLECTIONS

Grounding the card sort in previously collected study data made an important contribution to the effectiveness of the card sort exercise. The card sort statements were grounded in the study data, not only because they were based on the prior analysis of a large database but also because we used the women's own words as much as possible. Although we removed some cues to context, the statements remained closely connected to the women's experience—a connection that was evident from the emotion evoked by the statements. Identification with the statements facilitated rich think aloud data (Canter et al., 1985). Although some researchers (Weller, 1998) have expressed concern about the depth of information elicited by individual card sorts, our experience demonstrates the potential of this technique to generate rich qualitative data. Because the statements were evocative, the women needed time to deal with their emotions as well as to sort the cards. The 30 cards selected were manageable in the context of this study, although some researchers use as many as 50 or 60 cards (Olson & Morse, 1996; Spradley, 1979).

Women participating in the card sort interview responded positively to the experience. Indeed, all of the women expressed a willingness to participate in other stages of the study. The exercise helped many women to recognize that they were not alone in their caregiving struggle. As one woman said, "I'm not the only one feeling this way." Because they felt isolated as caregivers, participants valued the opportunity to help others in a similar situation by participating in the research. They repeatedly assured the interviewer that they hoped this research would make a difference to other caregivers: "If it helps others with their caregiving, I am glad to do it."

Women participating in the research interview were able to reflect on their caregiving experience. Opportunity for such reflection was rare because of their caregiving demands. For example, over the course of the card sort, one woman realized that she appreciated her daughter's doctor more than she had recognized previously. Several women became tearful in the interview as they recalled the support received from their family members.

One woman reflected on how her experience throughout the interview changed her perspective on the following statement: "I had to make sure my relative was getting the care needed." In the first card sort (an unconstrained sort), she said it was her responsibility to make sure that her relative was getting what she needed. In the second sort (constrained as helpful, unhelpful, and unclear), she placed the card in the helpful pile. When she did the third card sort (constrained as helpful or unhelpful), she said that this was a pronounced responsibility for her, as she did not have confidence in health professionals because they did not meet her relative's needs. Therefore, she placed this card in the unhelpful pile in the last card sort. This is consistent with the suggestion of others (Canter et al., 1985) that multiple card sorts might be a self-exploration process in which people revised their choices as they come to a fuller understanding of their conceptual systems or grow in their self-knowledge. This illustrates the importance of capturing the rationale for participant choices through recording their think aloud commentary.

Women also felt that the card statements could be used to teach family members and others about caregiving. One woman suggested that the card sort statements should be made into a board game that would stimulate conversation about caregiving among family members. Some women found it validating to have their experience of nonsupport aptly reflected in the statements. Similarly, other women said the statements would be helpful because they would inform others of the challenges of caregiving.

Useful conceptual insights arose from identification of differences in the women's interpretations of the card sort statements. For example, the statement "They brought over food," although helpful for some, was considered unhelpful by others, because the caregiver or care recipient was on a diet (e.g., diabetic diet) or the food was inappropriate because of the allergies of the care recipient or other family members. Similarly, the statement "The staff thought I was overprotective. They did not want to do as I asked." evoked negative emotions for many women, but others inferred that staff members understood their concern for their relative and sought what was in their best interest. Viewed in this way, the situation was seen as a learning opportunity for the caregiver.

The card sort was effective in eliciting detailed information about the types of nonsupport experienced by women in each caregiving situation because women often provided personal anecdotes to illustrate the statement on the card. When responding to a statement that depicted nonsupport generically, some women described what had been different and helpful in their own experience. Their anecdotes demonstrated the utility of using generic terms in the card sort statements. For example, one woman interpreted the statement that staff thought the caregiver was overprotective in the context of staff in a school setting, although the original statement came from a hospital setting. This was useful in expanding our knowledge of how similar issues occurred in slightly different ways and contexts for women in different caregiving situations. Some women did multiple interpretations of one card. To illustrate, one woman shared a story about a family member and another story about health professionals to illustrate the generic "they" in a card sort statement.

Data generated from the women's comments about their choices in the card sort enhanced our understanding of the basis for their decisions and the meaning of a statement for the woman. The women's comments revealed the expectations that they held for support from others and, in some cases, the source of their expectations. For example, one nurse noted a distinction between expectations for support that arose from the guidelines that were part of her experience in palliative care and oncology settings, and from her personal experience in caring for her husband who had cancer. Her comments indicated her awareness of a discrepancy between what was accepted in her professional role and what was experienced personally. This illustrates the value of attending to reflective comments or metastatements (Anderson & Jack, 1991) that indirectly reveal the categories a participant is using to monitor his or her thinking. Mothers of infants born prematurely sometimes responded to statements by differentiating between their initial and their current experience of nonsupport and support. They were particularly aware of changes in their caregiving situation as their infant's health improved, and they used this distinction in making their decisions.

CONCLUSION

We have described the practical challenges we experienced in designing and administering a card sort exercise in an ethnographic study of nonsupport and family caregiving. The strategies developed created a meaningful and manageable exercise and facilitated the participants' ability to complete the card sorts. The card sort exercise generated more detailed anecdotes and information about women's experience of nonsupport and support than we had anticipated. This data collection technique was useful in determining types of nonsupport that were experienced by women in diverse caregiving situations, identifying statements with variable interpretations, and understanding the women's rationale for labeling experiences as supportive or nonsupportive. Several conditions contributed to our positive experience with a card sort exercise, including systematic selection of content from a large preliminary data set, pilot exercises to examine the feasibility of the protocol and card sort statements, and interviewer warmth and sensitivity.

A valuable contribution of the card sort exercise was information about the variability in the meaning of similar interactions for different women and a beginning understanding of the criteria women used to make their decisions. The quality of data elicited through use of the card sort in this study exceeded our expectations and supports the merit of future research to refine the technique and explore its potential application in varied situations.

NOTE

Originally published in Neufeld, A., Harrison, M. J., Rempel, G., Larocque, S., Dublin, S., Stewart, M., & Hughes, K. (2004). Practical issues in using a card sort in a study of nonsupport and family caregiving. *Qualitative Health Research, 14*(10), 1418–1428.

REFERENCES

Anderson, K., & Jack, D. C. (1991). Learning to listen: Interview techniques and analysis. In S. Gluck& D. Patai (Eds.), *Women's words: The feminist practice of oral history* (pp. 11–26). New York: Routledge.

Beaver, K., Bogg, J., & Luker, K. A. (1999). Decision-making role preferences and information needs: A comparison of colorectal and breast cancer. *Health Expectations,* 2(4), 266–276.

Bernard, H. R. (2000). *Social research methods: Qualitative and quantitative approaches.* Thousand Oaks, CA: Sage.

Borgatti, S. P. (1999). Elicitation techniques for cultural domain analysis. In J. J. Schensul, M. D. LeCompte, B. K. Nastasi, & S. P. Borgatti (Eds.), *Enhanced ethnographic methods* (pp. 115–151). Walnut Creek, CA: Altamira.

Canter, D., Brown, J., & Groat, L. (1985). A multiple sorting procedure for studying conceptual systems. In M. Brenner, J. Brown, & D. Canter (Eds.), *The research interview: Uses and approaches* (pp. 79–114). London: Academic Press.

Caulkins, D. (1998). Consensus analysis: Do Scottish business advisers agree on models of success? In V. C. deMunck & E. J. Sobo (Eds.), *Using methods in the field: A practical introduction and casebook* (pp. 179–195). Walnut Creek, CA: Altamira.

Davison, B. J., & Degner, L. F. (1997). Empowerment of men newly diagnosed with prostate cancer. *Cancer Nursing, 20*, 187–196.

Johnson, J. C., & Griffith, D. C. (1998). Visual data: Collection, analysis and representation. In V. C. deMunck & E. J. Sobo (Eds.), *Using methods in the field: A practical introduction and casebook* (pp. 211–228). Walnut Creek, CA: Altamira.

Lang, F., & Carstensen, L. (2002). Time counts: Future time perspective, goals and social relationships. *Psychology and Aging, 17*(1), 125–139.

Luniewski, M., Reigle, J., & White, B. (1999). Card sort: An assessment tool for the educational needs of patients with heart failure. *American Journal of Critical Care, 8*(5), 297–302.

Miller, W. L., & Crabtree, B. F. (1999). Clinical research: A multimethod typology and qualitative roadmap. In B. F. Crabtree & W. L. Miller (Eds.), *Doing qualitative research* (pp. 3–30). Thousand Oaks, CA: Sage.

Morse, J. M., & Field, P. A. (1995). *Qualitative research methods for health professionals* (2nd ed.). Thousand Oaks, CA: Sage.

Nastasi, B. K., & Berg, M. J. (1999). Using ethnography to strengthen and evaluate intervention programs. In J. J. Schensul, M. D. LeCompte, G. A. Hess, B. K. Nastasi, M. J. Berg, L.Williamson, et al. (Eds.), *Using ethnographic data: Interventions, public programming, and public policy* (pp. 1–56). Walnut Creek, CA: Altamira.

Olson, K. L., & Morse, J. M. (1996). Explaining breast self-examination practice. *Health Care for Women International, 17*(6), 575–591.

Prus, R. (1996). *Symbolic interaction and ethnographic research*. Albany: State University of New York Press.

Rolland, J. S. (1990). Anticipatory loss: A family systems developmental framework. *Family Process, 29*(3), 229–244.

———. (1993). Mastering family challenges in serious illness and disability. In F. Walsh (Ed.), *Normal family processes* (pp. 444–473). New York: Guilford.

———. (1994). *Families, illness, and disability: An integrative treatment model*. New York: Basic Books.

Roos, G. (1998). Pile sorting: "Kids like candy." In V. C. deMunck & E. J. Sobo (Eds.), *Using methods in the field: A practical introduction and casebook* (pp. 97–110). Walnut Creek, CA: Altamira.

Ryan, G. W., & Bernard, H. R. (2000). Data management and analysis methods. In N. K. Denzin & Y. S. Lincoln (Eds.), *Handbook of qualitative research* (pp. 769–800). Thousand Oaks, CA: Sage.

Spradley, J. P. (1979). *The ethnographic interview*. New York: Holt, Rinehart and Winston.

Weller, S. C. (1998). Structured interviewing and questionnaire construction. In H. R. Bernard (Ed.), *Handbook of methods in cultural anthropology* (pp. 365–409). Walnut Creek, CA: Altamira.

Weller, S. C., & Romney, A. K. (1988). *Systematic data collection*. Newbury Park, CA: Sage.

11

Facilitating Participation of a Vulnerable Group: Immigrant Women

Feminist research has identified inadequacies in our knowledge of women's health. Inadequacies arise from the omission of issues important to women and the extrapolation to women of findings from research on men (Thorne & Varcoe, 1998). Knowledge of women's health is also restricted by the failure to include diverse groups of women in research. Although this is an important criterion of excellence in feminist research, it is often difficult to gain access to diversified samples (Reinharz, 1992). Moreover, there is little available information about the practical dimensions of research associated with including diverse groups of women from immigrant and minority ethnic and racial populations (e.g., Collins, 1990; hooks, 1981; Moraga & Anzaldua, 1981; Reinharz, 1992). The purpose of this chapter is to discuss issues related to the recruitment and participation of immigrant women in research.

Research on the health-related issues that immigrant women experience is an important priority. Immigrants and refugees are increasing in number in the United States (Lipson & Meleis, 1989), and in Canada, women comprise half of the total number of immigrants (Anderson, 1987; Statistics Canada, 1995). As a result of women's immigrant status, key determinants of their health, such as income and social support, are compromised (National Forum on Health, 1998), and women experience health risks associated with the increased stressors and loss of support that accompany migration and resettlement (Lipson & Meleis, 1989).

241

Immigrant women can experience cumulative negative effects on health status arising from migration and resettlement in combination with life transitions such as parenting or caring for elders (Meleis, Lipson, Muecke, & Smith, 1998). Within their households, gender roles may be reconfigured after immigration with the renegotiation of men's and women's work and income-sharing arrangements (Brettell & deBerjeois, 1992). Immigrant women consequently carry multiple roles, some of which are invisible, and deal with cultural differences in the symbolic meaning of interactions. These women may often confront disappointment as their life course fails to fulfill their cultural expectations (Meleis, 1991).

Health system reform and restructuring have been economically driven (Armstrong, 1996a) and not specifically sensitive to the needs of immigrant women, who must deal with potentially conflicting cultural values and patterns as well as face culture-related barriers in using health care services (Anderson, 1991). Studies have found that these women are especially ill-served when health and social services reduce the time allotted for professional-client encounters or increase the responsibility of family members (Spitzer, 2000). Furthermore, services and policies may lack cultural sensitivity, differentially restrict women's access to resources, fail to address the most pressing needs, or be seen as unacceptable by immigrant women (National Forum on Health, 1997; Stevens, 1993).

Exclusion of women from ethnic minorities in the collection of health and social science data further contributes to their marginalization and produces findings that are often unsuitable for a growing sector of the population. The inclusion of immigrant women as study participants is vital so that their voices can be heard and their concerns identified. The same characteristics that define their vulnerability to health risks and restrict their access to services also present barriers to their inclusion in research.

Although recruitment of immigrant women as study participants is known to be difficult, little is known about why this is so. There is inadequate information about successful, practical solutions that are acceptable to immigrant women. Those investigators who have addressed issues of research design (e.g., DeVault, 1995; Riessman, 1987) have focused on racial-ethnic dynamics in conducting and interpreting interviews rather than on the initial stages of research, when recruitment and access are critical issues. Edwards (1990) provides one detailed discussion of recruitment in a study on the education of Black women. In her study, standard techniques of recruiting were culturally inappropriate and thus largely ineffective. Her discussion, and this general gap in the literature, suggest that there is a great deal to be gained from considering issues of recruitment and participation in more detail, particularly as this is an essential first step in ensuring greater diversity in research populations.

In this chapter, we present issues related to recruitment and participation in our ethnographic study of South Asian and Chinese immigrant women in Canada who are caring for a family member with a chronic health problem or disability. We begin with a brief description of the methodology for the study. We then review feminist principles that guide participation of immigrant and ethnic populations in research and address the challenges we experienced. Our discussion concludes with reflection on our experience and that of other researchers.

STUDY OF IMMIGRANT WOMEN CAREGIVERS

The goal of our research was to understand the experience of Chinese and South Asian women family caregivers who are recent or past immigrants. The specific study objectives were (a) to identify the nature of the conditions within which these women give care, (b) to understand how and when they access informal sources of support, and (c) to examine their experience in accessing health and social service resources.

We used ethnographic inquiry to provide access to "in vivo" descriptions of the women's caregiving situations and their experience in obtaining support from family, friends, and community agencies. Incorporation of an interpretive critical perspective within ethnography (Morrow, 1994) focused attention on the cultural and structural conditions that are a source of power and control in the women's lives. This methodological orientation required consideration of systemic, institutional characteristics as well as the characteristics of individual women and their families. We sought to conduct the study from a feminist perspective that facilitated involvement of the women and minimized differences in social status and background (Reinharz, 1992). Our method differed from participatory feminist research or participatory action research because we did not incorporate the same depth and continuity of involvement of the women in constructing the research design (Maguire, 1987).

Caregiving situations included care of a disabled or developmentally delayed child and care of elderly parents or a spouse with a chronic illness. Each woman was interviewed once (n = 28), and some women (n = 12) participated in an in-depth case study. The case study included a participant observation visit and, in some cases, an interview with a person who assisted them with caregiving. The setting for the study was a medium-sized urban community in Western Canada, where a large percentage of the immigrant population was Chinese or South Asian.

GUIDING PRINCIPLES

Participation and recruitment of immigrant women in research can usefully be considered in the context of guiding principles within feminist research. We have been guided by the perspectives of Sandra Harding (1987), who argues that three key elements in feminist research include (a) starting with the experiences of diverse groups of women (i.e., developing questions from their lives), (b) engaging in research that benefits women in some way, and (c) placing the researcher and research process on the same critical plane as the overt subject matter so that all come under scrutiny. The adequacy of the understanding we can achieve through research is influenced by whom we include or exclude from the study and the nature of the questions we ask or fail to ask. To generate knowledge that is beneficial to immigrant women, we seek to raise questions about issues that the women themselves consider problematic. Knowledge will be perceived as beneficial when it includes an understanding of the nature of the external forces that shape the conditions of women's lives and how they may be changed. Information about influences on the researchers' perspectives (e.g., race, gender, class, and culture) and how they may have shaped the research endeavor is also necessary to enable women participants and others to evaluate the research findings. Although there is a risk that researchers who do not share the same social location or perspectives as immigrant women may reinforce current divisions, the exclusion of diverse groups of women helps to maintain existing power differentials (Edwards, 1990).

As others have argued, there is often a tension between the abstract presentation of feminist guiding principles and the practical options available in the research endeavor (Kelly, Burton, & Regan, 1994; Thorne & Varcoe, 1998). Central to this tension are issues of unequal power that are embedded in hierarchical relationships among researchers, research assistants, and participants in control over the research process and in the interpretation and distribution of findings (Wolf, 1996).

In this chapter, we discuss practical recruitment strategies we used in an attempt to reflect feminist guiding perspectives.

Access to the Experience of Diverse Groups of Women

We sought ways of involving immigrant women in determining the important issues to be addressed in the study and the most effective methods of initiating communication. In developing the proposal, we interviewed women staff members of relevant immigrant-serving and community agencies about the issues they considered important from the perspective of their personal and professional roles. Subsequent to receiving funding, we established an advisory committee. Members of the committee provided advice on approaches to recruitment and interviewing as well as feedback on recruitment materials and interview guides. The advisory committee included women who represented various mainstream, immigrant-serving, and ethno-specific community agencies. For example, we included representatives of agencies that provide home care, others that serve immigrant and refugee populations from any country of origin, Chinese and Indo-Canadian organizations, and individuals from the ethnic communities involved. The advisory committee helped us to identify suitable recruitment mechanisms. This approach provided limited opportunity for immigrant women and their advocates to influence the scope of the study in the initial stages. Use of an ethnographic approach enabled modification of the research method in response to the immigrant women's perspectives once the study was initiated. For example, the guiding questions for interviews were modified in response to feedback from the first immigrant women participants.

Within the Canadian context, the profile of the population of immigrant women is very diverse (Statistics Canada, 1995). To incorporate diversity, we sought to include women who were both recent and long-term immigrants as well as women from at least two different ethno-cultural groups. We included Chinese and South Asian women because they comprised a large percentage of immigrant women in the local geographic area. The percentage of immigrants coming to Canada from the Asia Pacific region was 45% in 1987 and has continued to increase (Chard, Badets, & Howatson, 2000).

We took the advice of women in the local ethnic communities to include women who viewed themselves as being of the same ethnic background but came from different countries. We therefore included women who immigrated from Pakistan, Sri Lanka, and India as well as women from Taiwan, Hong Kong, and mainland China. These geographic boundaries also provided some degree of homogeneity in women's previous experience. We considered recent immigrants to be those who had lived in Canada 7 years or less and long-term immigrants as those residing in Canada 15 years or more.

Women recruited in our study also varied in educational level, income, facility in English, and the immigration program under which they had entered Canada. These differences are characteristic of immigrant women in the Canadian context. Since 1976, applicants have entered Canada through either a family reunification or an independent immigration category that provided for entrance as skilled workers, business class entrepreneurs, or investors (Fleras & Eliott, 1999). Many of those who entered in the independent category subsequently applied for relatives to join them under the family reunification clause, which requires them to guarantee the provision of their relative's essential needs for several years and restricts access to some publicly funded programs, such as income security. Despite possessing higher education (Chard et al., 2000; Citizenship & Immigration Canada, 2009; Simmons, 1990) and being employed full-time more often, immigrant women and men have lower-than-average incomes compared to the Canadian-born population and are concentrated in administrative, clerical, sales, and service jobs (Beaujot & Rappak, 1990; Chard et al., 2000). In addition, in the past women immigrating to Canada often had less access than men to government-sponsored, English-language educational programs (Ng, 1993) although more recently, free language instruction has been made available through Citizenship and Immigration Canada to all adult family members (Citizenship and Immigration Canada, 2004; 2007).

Another adaptation in the study involved the recognition of cultural variations in the assignment of family caregiving responsibilities. The Euro-Canadian norm of an individual woman who provides care to a dependent family member did not fit many families in our study. Having a flexible methodology that allowed for in-depth interviews with other family members who participated in the caregiving enabled us to include some of these additional caregivers as participants and to recognize some of the cultural variations in caregiving arrangements. For instance, in one Chinese family in our study, the grandparents provided care to a disabled child until the parents were reunited with the family several years later.

Members of the advisory committee emphasized personal communication as the most effective mechanism for initiating contact with immigrant women. We found that key individuals within the ethnic communities helped to legitimize the project to women who were interested in participating. To identify key individuals, we employed research assistants of the same ethnic and language backgrounds as the women we sought for participation in the study. Personal communication between community members was also helpful. Some of the women interviewed subsequently referred other women to the study.

We also sought to contact women by advertising through ethnic community newspapers, newsletters of community organizations, and local radio announcements. Research assistants translated the required materials into the languages appropriate for clients of each participating agency. Immigrant-serving agencies with a multicultural mandate required materials that displayed all relevant languages, whereas others required materials only in the language of their ethnic group. For advertisements in Chinese, it was important that the Chinese research assistants record their Chinese name. We found, however, that advertising alone yielded few volunteers and that the women generally indicated that they had heard about the study through personal contacts.

Benefits for Immigrant Women

We sought to incorporate benefits for the women that were relevant to their caregiving situation and reduced the burden of participation. Although we considered providing reimbursement for interviews, we chose instead to provide information on access to community services for family caregivers. In part, our decision was influenced by the policy of the funding agency that did not permit honoraria for participants. The advisory group assisted us in selecting and assembling a package of information about relevant local resources. We verified that the information we included about each resource specified services currently available. For example, some agencies had insufficient staff resources to respond to individual requests for assistance but provided general information. Other agencies with larger staff resources provided detailed information on their services and the names of contact persons.

To reduce the burden on participants, the interview times and locations were flexible. Immigrant women selected the location for the interview, which was usually in their home, although some caregivers chose to be interviewed at a public location in the community. To encourage ease of communication, we provided the opportunity for women to speak in their first language, which almost half of the women (43%) did.

To give immigrant women caregivers the opportunity to meet other women in similar situations and a forum for expressing their views and recommendations on programs and policies, we offered focus groups conducted in their choice of language. Food and expenses for child care and transportation were covered. To further increase the benefit of the study for women, we included other focus groups for policy makers and program managers of mainstream and immigrant-serving agencies. These groups discussed the implications of study findings for policies and programs and identified advocacy initiatives that benefit immigrant women.

Placing the Researcher and Research Process on the Same Level

Attempting to reduce the power differential that may exist between immigrant women and researchers is important to enable the voices of immigrant women to be heard. When the research process itself reinforces existing divisions, the political nature of the personal experience of diverse groups of women is unrecognized. In this study, the team of investigators comprised women who are culturally of Euro-Canadian backgrounds and research assistants from the ethnic communities, who functioned as cultural brokers. Research assistants who act as cultural brokers can help to reduce the power differential that may exist between the researchers and immigrant women by facilitating opportunities for women to describe their personal experiences in a context in which cultural nuances can be recognized. As cultural brokers, research assistants also sensitize the investigators to perspectives that would otherwise be unrecognized. We acknowledge that power differentials between researchers and immigrant women are replicated in our relationships with the research assistants/cultural brokers. These relationships are inscribed not only by cultural difference and its attendant privileges but also by age, educational level, and academic position. We attempted to ameliorate these structural inequities by placing ourselves in the role of learners and by trying to remain responsive to the advice of the research assistants. Research assistants met regularly with the principal investigator and attended advisory committee meetings.

Participation in the study also provided some benefits for research assistants. They had an opportunity to gain new skills as well as a part-time salary. For example, they received training in interviewing and learned the skills involved in the recruitment and coordination of a research study. For those who were graduate and undergraduate students, these skills are important for research assistants' ongoing studies and future careers. While working with faculty members who are active researchers, student assistants gained access to mentorship with accompanying support and information relevant to their careers. Involvement in the study is also useful for research assistants who are not students. The skills and experience they acquire are transferable to other situations and can create new employment opportunities.

The linguistic diversity of the South Asian and Chinese communities offered additional challenges. Written materials, such as recruitment posters and consent forms, were translated into several languages. We also sought to provide an opportunity for immigrant women to be interviewed in the language of their choice. This was possible because the research assistants were fluent in the languages of the participants. Communication in the participant's language of choice was an advantage, as women may be reluctant to speak of their personal experience through an interpreter, particularly if the only available person is a male relative. The research assistants conducting the interviews translated those that were conducted in a language other than English. Research assistants helped to interpret aspects of the cultural context important in understanding the participant's intended meaning and attached a memo to the interview transcript documenting this information. They also reviewed the transcripts of interviews and made corrections as needed or provided additional explanatory comments. We employed these strategies to assist us in interpreting the meaning of the interview data and in understanding cultural variations. We held regular meetings with the research assistants to discuss progress in data collection and to make any necessary adjustments. These meetings were an important opportunity for debriefing and promoted supportive interaction among the interviewers. In addition, their participation in meetings of the advisory committee facilitated dialogue with committee members because they had a detailed understanding of the cultural context and issues within the ethnic communities.

The tasks of translation and interpretation require different skills, although the distinction is often overlooked (Spitzer, Henry, & Popp, 1998). The complexities of intercultural understanding and transfer are not readily captured by the use of a literal translation and back translation. When the focus is cultural transfer, the translator can focus on the meaning of the text in the target language and the way in which the information is received. The role of bicultural and multilingual research assistants conversant in Mandarin, Cantonese, Punjabi, Urdu, and Hindi who possess skills as translators and interpreters facilitated this communication in our study. Their relationship with the remainder of the research team ensured that issues of translation and interpretation remained an iterative process.

DISCUSSION

The issues we confronted in relation to sampling and recruitment required complex strategies developed within the context of a specific site (Arcury & Quandt, 1999). The issues and associated strategies were influenced by academic, funding, and community agency expectations. Because researchers were located within a university setting, the research was embedded in the context of university expectations in relation to academic credibility, methods of conducting research in the community, ethical guidelines, and the demands of other aspects of faculty members' roles. The research was also subject to the policies and agenda of the funding agency that determined the allocation of funds, salary scales, reporting periods, and roles of investigators.

Within the local setting, mainstream and immigrant-serving agencies that collaborated with us in conducting the study were seeking useful information to guide the development and delivery of services that would assist immigrant women. Immigrant women participating in the study indicated that they were motivated to participate because they were hopeful that sharing their experience would be useful in helping others in similar situations and in improving available resources. Cost cutting and restructuring in the health care sector were prevalent in the local situation (Armstrong, 1996b; Hughes, Lowe, & McKinnon, 1996). Within this context of varied expectations by university, funding, and community agencies, as well as by participants, the goal of the research was to contribute to both theoretical and practical knowledge.

In seeking to involve a diverse group of immigrant women and work within the guidelines of feminist principles, we confronted challenges in attracting immigrant women and in interacting with the women in ways that established trust and were culturally sensitive. We next reflect on our experience and the experience of other researchers in addressing these challenges.

Connecting with Immigrant Women of Diverse Characteristics

Our first challenge was to identify immigrant women with whom to interact in relation to the goals of the study. Traditional criteria for diversity of immigrant populations provided some direction for the selection of the study sample, but there was little information available to guide us in differentiating meaningful subgroups of women. Recognition of subgroups, however, is important in developing culturally sensitive programs. In addition, the characteristics of immigrant women have implications for the recruitment process as well as for the study. Immigrant women who have been in their new country longer may be more easily recruited because they have greater facility in English and are more likely to access health care services. Because they have greater facility in English, they may also be more likely to respond to information in the public media (Braun, Takamura, & Mougeot, 1996; Tabora & Flaskerud, 1997). Recruitment strategies that use advertising and recruitment through health care agencies may therefore bias the sample toward women who are long-term residents. This occurs because higher levels of acculturation are associated with a greater use of health care services. Cultural background and country of origin may also influence recruitment. For example, because individuals from Asian communities may underutilize services for parents (Harachi, Catalano, & Hawkins, 1997) or caregivers (Braun et al., 1996), recruitment through community agencies may limit the number of Asian women included.

Development of a network of key individuals and agencies in the community and the use of snowball sampling facilitated referrals of potential study participants. Although these are traditional approaches in ethnographic and qualitative research, there are limitations that should be acknowledged. Faugier and Sargeant (1997) noted that recruitment methods involving some form of personal referral assume a linkage or bond with other individuals in the sample. As a consequence, the sample will include subsets of individuals with a connection to each other and overlapping circles of acquaintance. This approach reduces the likelihood of including those more socially distant from the key informants and increases the probability that well-known or popular individuals will more often be included. To address this limitation, we sought to work with individuals from distinct personal and professional networks. We accomplished this by establishing an advisory committee with diverse representation from a range of mainstream and immigrant-serving community agencies and by employing three research assistants, each of whom was affiliated with a different community.

Engaging Women in Culturally Sensitive Ways

We employed three approaches to foster trust and enhance cultural sensitivity. These included emphasizing personal communication, employing research assistants from ethnic communities, and interviewing women in their first language. The value of personal communication was emphasized by members of our advisory committee and is well recognized as a key mechanism for engaging members of minority or hard-to-reach populations. Personal contact may help to alleviate the skepticism of some potential participants who are distrustful of official agencies such as the university. In a Middle Eastern immigrant population, individuals were distrustful of research and of the university, which they associated with the government (Lipson & Meleis, 1989). Edwards (1990) had a similar experience in recruiting Black women through the distribution of letters of invitation by the educational institution where they were registered as students. In our research, this seemed to be less of a problem, perhaps because of our affiliations with immigrant-serving and ethnic community agencies. Other researchers (Cannon, Higginbotham, & Leung, 1988) attribute the preference for direct-contact methods to women's need for personal assurance that the research is worthwhile, will not have a negative impact, and maintains anonymity and confidentiality.

We sought to increase trust and diminish the power differential between researchers and immigrant women by employing research assistants from the ethnic communities. There are differing views on the conditions that are most effective in fostering trust (Reinharz, 1992). Some argue that the anonymity and social distance present in interaction with a stranger may facilitate disclosure more than interaction with someone who is a member of the same community because of a greater threat to privacy and confidentiality. Others emphasize the importance of establishing a close relationship with participants prior to initiating the research process. Like Meleis (1991), we found that the employment of research assistants who were familiar with the women's communities and languages was beneficial and increased the likelihood that participants would feel confident in sharing their experiences.

Research assistants from the ethnic communities can assist researchers to make culturally appropriate interpretations of participants' comments and descriptions of their experiences. We learned that the terms *caregiving* and *barriers* were inappropriate for Chinese women in relation to caring for a relative. We therefore needed to take into account the hesitation of Chinese immigrant women to discuss caregiving and the illness or disability of relatives. Other researchers (Dowling & Weiner, 1997; Hinton, Guo, Hillygus, & Levkoff, 2000) reported difficulty in recruiting Chinese caregivers, as they considered it bad luck to discuss illness, felt shame in having a "damaged" relative, or considered symptoms such as dementia-related changes as part of normal aging. Chinese women did not want outsiders to know about their family member's weakness. To avoid negative connotations or implications of blame, our interview questions also asked the immigrant women about what helps them to give care. This is consistent with an approach used by others that focuses instead on strengths and a continuum of supportiveness (Massat & Lundy, 1997). Research assistants also assisted us with culturally appropriate interpretation of the interview data. Riessman (1987) illustrates the importance of this role. In her study, one interviewer failed to understand a Hispanic participant's culturally influenced thematic account of her marital experience. The interviewer attempted unsuccessfully to document the participant's experience from a chronological rather than a thematic perspective. Observation and interpretation of nonverbal language and omissions are also dependent on cultural knowledge (Matsuoka, 1993). To facilitate this aspect of the research, research assistants maintained detailed field notes for each interview. Matsuoka noted the importance of the cultural meaning of nonverbal language and omissions in research with ethnic elders. There may also be cultural variability in the acceptability of communicating personal feelings about experience. For example, it may be inappropriate to express emotions or a negative view. In one study of Japanese American women (Trockman et al., 1997), participants always balanced a negative statement with a positive one.

Membership of the research assistant in the same ethnic group as study participants does not ensure homogeneity. There may be important social, religious, economic, and educational divisions and differences that make the research assistant unacceptable to some participants or limit the degree of trust that can be established (Dyck, Lynam, & Anderson, 1995). It is helpful, therefore, for researchers to have access to an advisory committee or consultant familiar with the communities involved to identify such potential divisions, and either recruit staff who will be acceptable to subgroups or develop strategies to overcome potential barriers to their acceptance.

Although research assistants play an important role as cultural brokers in enhancing participant trust and culturally appropriate interpretation of data, they occupy an "in-between" position as mediators (Dyck et al., 1995). If research assistants have not had a personal opportunity to participate in the formulation of interview questions, they may question the suitability of the interview (Dyck et al., 1995) and find it difficult to respond to participants' criticisms (Phoenix, 1994). For example, research assistants encouraged us to modify questions about difficulties in caring for a relative. They suggested we first address what was "satisfying" but not as "what was the best part," as we had originally proposed. Their advice was based on the concern of Chinese participants that caring for a relative was expected and should not be viewed as a burden.

Practical Implications

Practical implications include the increased time and varied skills required to adapt recruitment materials in several languages, to establish and maintain connections with multiple immigrant-serving and community agencies, and to facilitate regular meetings with an advisory committee. Transcription and management of data is more time-consuming because interview guides must be adapted for each language, and interviews conducted in a language other than English must be translated and subsequently checked against the tape by someone familiar with the language. Languages involved in this study included Cantonese, Mandarin, Punjabi, and English. To connect effectively with different groups, it is necessary to employ a team of research assistants who collectively possess the required characteristics, including the ability to interview in two languages. This increases time in recruitment, training, and communication with research assistants, but it may enhance their ability to support each other. The investigative team included members with experience in working with immigrant women as well as in the content focus of the research (e.g., support of women family caregivers). The multidisciplinary research team members were from nursing, women's studies, sociology, anthropology, and health promotion. In our previous studies of women caregivers (Harrison & Neufeld, 1997; Neufeld & Harrison, 1995), we successfully recruited women through advertisement in community newspapers and health care agencies. These studies did not include an ethnically diverse group of women, nor did we work with an advisory committee. In another study, we employed research assistants with facility in another language, and interviews were conducted in another language and translated back into English (Stewart et al., 2001). The complexity of the present project necessitated extensive time and resources for recruitment of immigrant women participants from different countries of origin, communication with immigrant-serving agencies, orientation of research assistants, translation of interviews, and interpretation of cultural implications during data analysis.

CONCLUSION

Feminist research has expanded our understanding of women's lives, particularly as diversity among women has begun to receive the attention it deserves. It has also provided a rich and thought-provoking debate about the epistemological and methodological principles guiding research. Less developed, however, have been discussions about the practical research strategies needed to implement these principles and to ensure that diverse groups of women are included. There is a need for more sustained discussion around practical research strategies.

Our purpose therefore in this article was to contribute to an understanding of this important dimension of feminist research. Following Harding's (1987) guiding principles—particularly the commitment to reflexivity in the research process—we discussed the concrete research strategies developed in our study of immigrant women caregivers and evaluated the relative success and implications of these strategies. Our discussion highlights specific innovations we developed in research with diverse groups of women around issues of recruitment, trust, and cultural sensitivity. It also explicates the demands these innovations have placed on research team relationships, research time, and project resources. By sharing our experience, we hope to offer concrete strategies that may be helpful to other researchers and contribute to a deeper understanding of practical strategies for achieving diversity in research. We also hope to spark further discussion and debate on the important practical dimensions of doing feminist research.

NOTE

Originally published in Neufeld, A., Harrison, M. J., Hughes, K., Spitzer, D., & Stewart, M. (2001). Participation of immigrant women family caregivers in qualitative research. *Western Journal of Nursing Research, 23*(6), 575–591.

REFERENCES

Anderson, J. M. (1987). Migration and health: Perspectives on immigrant women. *Sociology of Health and Illness, 9*(4), 410–438.

———. (1991). Immigrant women speak of chronic illness: The social construction of the devalued self. *Journal of Advanced Nursing, 16*(6), 710–717.

Arcury, T., & Quandt, S. (1999). Participant recruitment for qualitative research: A site-based approach to community research in complex societies. *Human Organization, 58*(2), 128–141.

Armstrong, P. (1996a). Resurrecting "the family," interring "the state." *Journal of Comparative Family Studies, 27,* 221–247.

———. (1996b) Unraveling the safety net: Transformations in health care and their impact on women. In Janine Brodie (Ed.), *Women and Canadian public policy* (pp. 129–149). Toronto: Harcourt Brace.

Beaujot, R., & Rappak, J. P. (1990). The evolution of immigrant cohorts. In S. Halli, F. Trovato, & L. Drieger (Eds.), *Ethnic demography: Canadian immigrant, racial, and cultural variations* (pp. 111–140). Ottawa, ON: Carleton University Press.

Braun, K. L., Takamura, J. C., & Mougeot, T. (1996). Perceptions of dementia, caregiving, and help-seeking among recent Vietnamese immigrants. *Journal of Cross-Cultural Gerontology, 11,* 213–228.

Brettell, C., & deBerjeois, P. (1992). Anthropology and the study of immigrant women. In D. Gabaccia (Ed.), *Seeking common ground: Multidisciplinary studies of immigrant women in the United States* (pp. 41–63). Westport, CT: Greenwood.

Cannon, L. W., Higginbotham, E., & Leung, M. L. A. (1988). Race and class bias in qualitative research on women. *Gender and Society, 2*(4), 449–462.

Chard, J., Badets, J., & Howatson, L. (2000). Immigrant women. In M. Almey, S. Besserer, J. Chard, C. Lindsay, J. Normand, V. Pottie Bunge, H. Tait, & N. Zukewich (Eds.), *Women in Canada 2000: A gender-based statistical report* (Statistics Canada No. 89-503-XPE, pp.189–217). Ottawa, ON: Statistics Canada.

Citizenship & Immigration Canada. (2004). *Evaluation of the language instruction for newcomers to Canada (LINC) program.* Retrieved June 11, 2009, from http://www.cic.gc.ca/english/resources/evaluation/linc

———. (2007). *Welcome to Canada: What you should know.* Retrieved June 11, 2009, from http://www.cic.gc.ca/english/resources/publications/welcome

———. (2009). *Sponsoring your family.* Ottawa: Minister of Citizenship, Immigration and Multiculturalism: Canada. Retrieved June 11, 2009, from http://www.cic.gc.ca/english/immigrate/sponsor

Collins, P. H. (1990). *Black feminist thought: Knowledge, consciousness, and the politics of empowerment.* London: Routledge.

DeVault, M. (1995). Ethnicity and expertise: Racial-ethnic knowledge in sociological research. *Gender and Society, 9*(5), 612–631.

Dowling, G. A., & Weiner, C. L. (1997). Roadblocks encountered in recruiting patients for a study of sleep disruption in Alzheimer's disease. *Image: Journal of Nursing Scholarship, 29*(1), 59–64.

Dyck, I., Lynam, J., & Anderson, J. (1995).Women talking: Creating knowledge through differences in cross-cultural research. *Women's Studies International Forum, 18*(5), 611–626.

Edwards, R. (1990). Connecting method and epistemology. *Women's Studies International Forum, 13*(5), 477–490.

Faugier, J., & Sargeant, M. (1997). Sampling hard-to-reach populations. *Journal of Advanced Nursing, 26*, 790–797.

Fleras, A., & Eliott, J. L. (1999). *Unequal relations.* Scarborough, ON: Prentice Hall, Allyn & Bacon.

Harachi, T. W., Catalano, R. F., & Hawkins, J. D. (1997). Effective recruitment for parenting programs within ethnic minority communities. *Child and Adolescent Social Work Journal, 14*(1), 23–39.

Harding, S. (1987). Is there a feminist method? In S. Harding (Ed.), *Feminism and methodology* (pp. 1–14). Bloomington: Indiana University Press.

Harrison, M. J., & Neufeld, A. (1997). Women's experience of barriers to support while caregiving. *Health Care for Women International, 18*, 591–602.

Hinton, L., Guo, Z., Hillygus, J., & Levkoff, S. (2000).Working with culture: A qualitative analysis of barriers to the recruitment of Chinese American family caregivers for dementia research. *Journal of Cross-Cultural Gerontology, 15*, 119–137.

hooks, b. (1981). *Ain't I a woman?: Black women and feminism.* Boston: South End.

Hughes, K. D., Lowe, G. S., & McKinnon, A. L. (1996). Public attitudes toward budget cuts in Alberta: Biting the bullet or feeling the pain? *Canadian Public Policy, 22*(3), 268–284.

Kelly, L., Burton, S., & Regan, L. (1994). Researching women's lives or studying women's oppression? Reflections on what constitutes feminist research. In M. Maynard & J. Peters (Eds.), *Researching women's lives from a feminist perspective* (pp. 27–48). London: Taylor & Cranas.

Lipson, J. C., & Meleis, A. I. (1989). Methodological issues in research with immigrants. *Medical Anthropology, 12*, 103–115.

Maguire, P. (1987). *Doing participatory research: A feminist approach.* Amherst: University of Massachusetts Press.

Massat, C. R., & Lundy, M. (1997). Empowering research participants. *Affilia, 12*(1), 33–56.

Matsuoka, A. K. (1993). Collecting qualitative data through interviews with ethnic older people. *Canadian Journal on Aging, 12*(3), 216–233.

Meleis, A. I. (1991). Between two cultures: Identity, roles, and health. *Health Care for Women International, 12*, 365–377.

Meleis, A. I., Lipson, J., Muecke, M., & Smith, G. (1998). *Immigrant women and their health: An olive paper.* Indianapolis, IN: Sigma Theta Tau International.

Moraga, C., & Anzaldua, G. (1981). *This bridge called my back: Writings by radical women of color.* New York: Kitchen Table Women of Color.

Morrow, R. (1994). *Critical theory and methodology.* Thousand Oaks, CA: Sage.

National Forum on Health. (1997). *Canada health action: Building on the legacy.* Ottawa, ON: Author.

———. (1998). *Canada health action: Building on the legacy: Vol. 2. Determinants of health: Adults and seniors.* Ottawa, ON: Author.

Neufeld, A., & Harrison, M. J. (1995). Reciprocity and social support in caregivers' relationships: Variations and consequences. *Qualitative Health Research, 5*, 349–366.

Ng, R. (1993). Racism, sexism, and immigrant women. In S. Burt, L. Code, & L. Dorney (Eds.), *Changing patterns: Women in Canada* (pp. 279–308). Toronto, ON: McClelland & Stewart.

Phoenix, A. (1994). Practising feminist research: The intersection of gender and "race" in the research process. In M. Maynard & J. Purvis (Eds.), *Researching women's lives from a feminist perspective* (pp. 49–69). London: Taylor and Francis.

Reinharz, S. (1992). *Feminist methods in social research*. New York: Oxford University Press.

Riessman, C. (1987). When gender is not enough: Women interviewing women. *Gender and Society, 1*(2), 172–207.

Simmons, A. (1990). New wave immigrants: Origins and characteristics. In S. Halli, F. Trovato, & L. Drieger (Eds.), *Ethnic demography: Canadian immigrant, racial, and cultural variations* (pp. 141–159). Ottawa, ON: Carleton University Press.

Spitzer, D. (2000). They don't listen to your body: Minority women, nurses, and childbirth. In D. Gustafson (Ed.), *Care and consequences: Women and health reform* (pp. 85–106). Halifax, NS: Fernwood.

Spitzer, D., Henry, C., & Popp, J. (1998). Back to basics: Towards a consensus on health translation. *Health and Cultures, 13*(2), 5–6.

Statistics Canada. (1995). *Women in Canada: A statistical report* (3rd ed.). Ottawa, ON: Statistics Canada Housing, Family and Social Statistics Division.

Stevens, S. (1993). *Community-based programs for a multicultural society: A guidebook for service providers*, Winnipeg, MB: Planned Parenthood Manitoba.

Stewart, M., Hart, G., Mann, K., Langille, L., Jackson, S., & Reidy, M. (2001). Telephone support group intervention for hemophiliacs with HIV/AIDS and their family caregivers. *International Journal of Nursing Studies, 28*(2), 209–225.

Tabora, B. L., & Flaskerud, J. H. (1997). Mental health beliefs, practices, and knowledge of Chinese American immigrant women. *Issues in Mental Health Nursing, 18*, 173–189.

Thorne, S., & Varcoe, C. (1998). The tyranny of feminist methodology in women's health research. *Health Care for Women International, 19*, 481–493.

Trockman, C. T., Murdaugh, C., Kadohiro, J. K., Petrovitch, H., Curb, J. D., & White, L. (1997). Adapting instruments for caregiver research in elderly Japanese American women. *Journal of Cross-Cultural Gerontology, 12*, 109–120.

Wolf, D. L. (1996). Situating feminist dilemmas in fieldwork. In D. Wolf (Ed.), *Feminist dilemmas in fieldwork* (pp. 1–55). Boulder, CO: Westview.

Index

Note: An f or t following a page number indicates a figure or a table, respectively.